C000298694

# CHOOSING
# TO STAY

## HOW CANCER GAVE ME MY LIFE BACK

## MO HAQUE

# RETHINK PRESS

First published in Great Britain 2018 by Rethink Press
(www.rethinkpress.com)

© Copyright Momenul Haque

All rights reserved. No part of this publication may be reproduced, stored in or introduced into a retrieval system, or transmitted, in any form, or by any means (electronic, mechanical, photocopying, recording or otherwise) without the prior written permission of the publisher.

The right of Momenul Haque to be identified as the author of this work has been asserted by him in accordance with the Copyright, Designs and Patents Act 1988.

This book is sold subject to the condition that it shall not, by way of trade or otherwise, be lent, resold, hired out, or otherwise circulated without the publisher's prior consent in any form of binding or cover other than that in which it is published and without a similar condition including this condition being imposed on the subsequent purchaser.

Cover image © Marc Garcia @marcgarcia.ldn

# CONTENTS

To my nephews: Arfan, Ejaz, Aayan, Nuhan and Syam. You boys mean the world to me. I hope to see you all become men.

# INTRODUCTION

As I begin to write, my cancer story continues to develop day by day. I have no idea how it will end. I trust an appropriate ending will emerge, whatever the latest chapter in my life.

In fact, the emotional journey this book promises to be is like a metaphor for cancer: full of uncertainty. If I wait for the perfect time to write, I will never begin, so here goes – and the truth is, the story will continue even after this book comes to an end.

Let's begin.

The word 'cancer' is loaded with emotion, with fear, with sadness and, for many, with loss. For those with the disease, there is the loss of a regular way of living, a loss of dignity at times. For those who are caring for someone with the disease, there is a different set of challenges: seeing someone suffer is never easy. And then there are those who have experienced the death of a loved one. The word 'cancer' has so many painful connotations based on our previous experience.

Life changes after a cancer diagnosis – it certainly changed for me. Little things all of a sudden made a huge difference: a serious diagnosis gives life a new level of meaning, and for me, while death breathed closer than ever, paradoxically, I felt more alive than before.

In the first of the two sections in this book, I present the choices I made while I was at the mercy of doctors, facing what was ahead of me. With a grim outlook and 'the small chance' of survival I had been given, there seemed to be very little choice. 'What's the point of even having treatment?' was a question I asked myself.

Yet I found I was making choices every day, every moment. I now know we are making choices all the time, whether we are conscious of it or not, even when those choices are limited by cancer. Having no choice is no way to live a life, but believing another way is possible can be very tough. I still believe that with a bit of help, even in the most dire of circumstances, we can make effective choices. When we become aware that there is choice in every moment, there is a sense of liberation. 'Do I choose to stay?' became my primary question. It kept me going, and continues to do so to this very day.

As I revisit the choices I made in the lead-up to my diagnosis, during my treatment, and then a year later, when I heard the words 'there's nothing more we can do for you', I share my cancer story: a story of pain, of meaning, of turmoil, but also a story of hope.

In the second section I share the lessons I learned from the choices I made: lessons on how to live life when you've been given a life sentence, on how to keep hoping when there seems to be no hope left, on how to be vulnerable, on how to step out of your comfort zone again and again, on how to ask for and receive help. These lessons have given me a new framework for living my life in the context of the challenges I face every single day.

# SECTION ONE

# CHOICES

# CHOICE ONE

# CHALLENGES

In the summer of 2012, I was in a great place. I was at the peak of my health, and I was looking for a new challenge, a new way to stretch myself. London had just hosted the Olympic Games, and I was inspired to push for my own personal gold.

A challenge such as running a marathon seemed an easy option. I mean, running was something I did for fun. I also knew I had the cardio stamina to cycle for as long as I wanted, even though my mountain bike was collecting rust. But when it came to swimming, I was a novice. Training for a triathlon was a thought that inspired me. It would be the ultimate test. The first step was to learn to swim properly, so I joined a swimming club and began taking lessons in the early hours each Saturday.

Sport has always been a huge part of my life. As a kid I fell in love with football and cricket, but the 100m was the event I was best at, and I even dreamed of becoming an Olympic gold medallist, although that dream ended at the age of 11 when a PE teacher with a stop watch said my 13-second sprint was two seconds too slow. He wasn't going to pass me on to a specialist coach. As I became an adult, I discovered a love of long distance running. I would run 10km, three times a week, for fun. Running allowed me to forget everything: the politics at work, the drama in my life, and all the suffering on a global level that I heard on the news.

When I began studying sociology at college, my desire to make a difference in the world grew. Studying sociology and psychology, at university, back in 2001, was my way of better understanding the world and its people. I hoped I would find a meaningful career to eventually make that difference.

As my time at university drew to a close, my text books zapped the last remaining drops of my enthusiasm. Sociology, in a nutshell, taught me that society was fixed and inequality was deeply ingrained in a capitalist system that depended on a rich vs poor divide. There was an embedded hierarchy: the people who controlled the economy, education, law and order, politics and media did so to keep things the way they were. The interpretation I took was that 'the rich get richer, the poor get poorer'. I had very little hope left.

But then life has a funny way of dealing its hand.

I discovered the students' union in my final year of my studies, and I found a way to channel my energy for the much-needed change in the world I desired. I decided to run for Vice President. It was one of the most nerve-racking things I'd ever done in my 21 years up until that point, standing in front of audiences, asking students to vote for me because I wanted to make the world better, cleaner and fairer. Miraculously, from knowing no one in the SU, I became elected to one of the most influential student roles in the university. I got to attend meetings with the Vice Chancellor, as well as regular catch-ups with the Chief Finance Officer. It was one of the major achievements in my early career, and definitely one to add to my CV.

But things didn't go quite as I imagined. As my one-year term came to an end in 2005, I felt like a failure. It was the toughest year of my life. I was a lousy politician and I couldn't do any of the things I wanted. The people who controlled the finances in the higher echelons of the university could veto any decision, and they did. The students who had voted for me weren't happy in the slightest and made this known.

The lessons I learned in sociology appeared to be right. The system was too big for the changes I wanted. I was ready to resign when Dave, a fellow Vice President, said, 'Mo, if you run away from this, you'll be running your entire life.' Something resonated in those words, the impact of which I would, later in life, come to appreciate. I chose to stay to face, and survive, a dreaded 'vote of no confidence' motion.

## LIFE WAS TO DEAL A NEW HAND

As that year came to an end, an HR bulletin was sent around listing some courses that were taking place on campus. Optimum Health and Wellbeing was the one that grabbed my attention. It was just what I needed and I signed up. We practised mindfulness, yoga, a lot of introspection, and we were given a workbook to write down our thoughts and wellness plans. Going through the workbook, I read a quote from Tony Robbins (a life and business strategist): 'All personal breakthroughs happen with a change in belief'.

I had a flashback to when I was a teenager and saw Tony Robbins on TV commercials. 'Change your life in seven days' was his promise, and famous sports stars, actors and world leaders shared testimonials on how Tony had helped them reach the top of their game. I remembered my dream of being a champion, but also remembered my doubts as a kid: 'Who am I to aspire to be an Olympic gold medallist? What would people think of me listening to motivational tapes?' Then, as an adult, I contemplated how differently things might have turned out. 'Maybe he has a book?' – this new thought crossed my mind.

That is the story of how I got into the personal development industry, and found myself in the self-help sections of bookstores and seminar rooms around the world. Tony Robbins had published three books at the time. The first I read was Notes From A Friend, and it changed my life – no overstatement. Where sociology left me with no hope, this little gem was filled with inspirational story after inspirational story. How Viktor Frankl survived concentration camps, how Honda became a global brand following several set-backs, and how individuals like myself could take control of our future. 'If you ask a better question, you'll get a better answer' became a mantra for me. I began obsessing about asking better questions.

As I learned a new model for living, I affirmed that I would make this information accessible and available to students and young people. A new world was possible, and I wanted students to be at the forefront of change. It was a quest for knowledge, for wisdom, with the intention of sharing. And that is what I did. I began my career in student development, working in a university environment for the next decade, helping students to become leaders and change makers.

In my quest for continuous and never-ending improvement, I studied more books, listened to lectures and attended courses around the world. Tony Robbins led to Wayne Dyer, to Deepak Chopra, to Marianne Williamson, to John Demartini and many more. As I continued to immerse myself in self-development, I discovered new names and younger teachers closer to my age, such as Gabby B.

The year of the London Olympics was a great year of change for me. I had been associated with Middlesex University since 2001, initially as a student, and then as a member of staff. My department was going through its second major restructure since I joined, and I decided to call an end to my time there. I realised that if I stayed on, I'd be there for the rest of my career. It was an opportunity to try something new. I was already working on my triathlon goals by learning to swim, and I felt ready to take my career to a different environment.

Towards the end of 2012, I joined Kingston University, again working in student development. I grew accustomed to a new role, within a new team, working for a new organisation, and I enjoyed the challenges and the opportunities to explore other areas of work, especially in equality and diversity.

As the year 2014 progressed, things weren't so great anymore.

Health-wise, running was no longer easy. My times were off by several minutes, my 5k runs were minutes slower, and my 10k runs some 10 minutes longer. The triathlon idea was a distant memory and waking up on a Saturday morning for a swim was the last thing on my mind. At work, there was another restructure taking place, the third that I was involved in within a decade. Once again, I saw staff grow uncertain about their job security. Restructures aren't fun as people inevitably lose jobs, fear of which fuels gossip and speculation, and a culture emerges that runs counter to one of fulfilment.

I was working on a diversity project, for which I had applied and received a substantial amount of funding – more than £30,000. Yet the project's processes had me questioning my identity. The project was aimed at making university life accessible to students from certain deprived backgrounds. As I immersed myself in the project I realised that I was that very student as I was growing up – a Bangladeshi boy, classed as an ethnic minority, from a single-parent household (my dad died when I was two), my family on benefits. I received free school meals, and the school I attended was an inner city comprehensive, which was in Ofsted special measures and under constant scrutiny. These were some of the criteria used to target disadvantaged kids, and I was heavily involved. There were committees in place that aimed to make higher education a reality for kids just like myself. This project triggered a number of questions about who I was. I was labelled a disadvantaged kid while growing up, without even recognising it. 'Was I a disadvantaged kid? Did this affect my early life experiences and opportunities?' These became new questions for me. As I looked over my short professional life, and how decisions were made in the board rooms, I reminisced how the system was just how the sociology text books had described. With my identity shaken to the core, I became vulnerable. I began to break down in meetings as people made decisions about people like me. I struggled to articulate my thoughts and now, in my thirties, I felt inadequate.

I knew I didn't have the answers myself and found a group of diverse students who were passionate about finding solutions to problems they were encountering on campus and in society. I was in so much physical pain at this point, but this got me out of bed in the mornings and into work.

How life had changed in a matter of two years. That Olympic-inspired triathlon challenge was a distant memory as my physical health increasingly troubled me. Abdominal pain was taking over, and my mental health was shaky as I tried to understand my identity. It was one morning in October – the 24th, to be precise – in 2014 that the unbearable pain resulted in my going to hospital, and subsequently a new challenge awaited me.

## REFLECTION

It is clear that I have had challenges throughout my life, whether I chose them or not, or whether I was even aware of them. Yet there were always ways to overcome them, however painful they felt. This new physical pain was different: there was no explanation. I thought I had taken care of my body as well as I could, so the pain didn't make sense. Here was a new challenge that I couldn't simply run off.

CHOICE TWO

# TO STAY STRONG

I went to bed that night hoping the pain would magically have gone away in the morning. I didn't move one bit, I was glued to the same position, but the pain was so bad I found it difficult to breathe. After exchanging messages with my close friend Aadam, we decided the best thing for me to do was to go to A&E. Had my mother known earlier, she would have insisted I had gone the evening before. Reluctantly, I walked to A&E, a short distance from home, thinking about my workload. Another close friend, Sai, saw me from the bus. I must have looked terrible, because he sent me a message asking if I was okay.

At the hospital the nurse looked at me with a face that suggested I was wasting her time. 'Tummy ache, huh?' When I told her I hadn't taken any pain killers, she said, 'We feel pain, we take pain killers, and the pain goes away.' She proceeded to give me some tablets. I felt silly. I wondered whether it was that easy. I'd rather have been at work, anywhere but the hospital. In fact, I was working in between the waiting and all the tests I had that day. I took phone calls and was continually messaging my team. I was heavily involved in an important student diversity conference, student by-elections and strategy work. There was a lot to do.

The pain didn't go away with paracetamol as the nurse prophesised.

The doctor looked puzzled as the blood tests showed I was anaemic, which was unusual for 'a guy my age' (31). He said I would need to have cameras put inside me to find out what was going on at a later date. The chest x-ray and ECG (heart check) didn't show what might be wrong.

Over the course of the following six weeks, I had more hospital appointments, more blood tests, X-rays, and various types of scans. I continued to live with the pain, every moment of every day.

The tablets that I was given increased in potency: from paracetamol, to codeine, to cocodamol, to eventually the controlled tramadol. How I wished the nurse was right, but the pain wouldn't go away. I was struggling to sleep, but somehow managed to go to work during this time. I wasn't at my 100% best and was frustrated that I couldn't focus during a testing time. The elections came and went, the conference was a huge step forward into a detailed programme of activity ahead, yet I was finding it difficult to make it in to work each day.

It was now December and almost time for the dreaded cameras, but first I had an ultra sound scan. As I came out of the hospital following that scan, I was in tears. The scan didn't show anything to help detect the problem. I was overwhelmed, and the prospect of having cameras inserted didn't help. The bowel preparation laxatives didn't sound appealing either. The weight of being in continuous pain for six weeks was taking its toll.

My GP suggested I take some time off, so I booked a week off to allow for my endoscopy and colonoscopy procedures and the consultation appointment to find out the result. These procedures would entail a camera being inserted down my throat to see what was happening in the gastrointestinal tract, and another camera inserted through my bottom to examine any abnormalities in my colon.

## CAMERAS INSIDE

It was a Saturday afternoon and I was hungry following my bowel cleanse. The nurses did their thing: asked questions, completed forms and asked me to sign consent forms. All I wanted to know was whether the procedures would hurt. I was squeamish when they connected a cannula. I didn't like needles, and I have a history of nearly fainting at the sight of blood. Appropriately, I was sitting in a room set up for children. The posters on the wall were of cartoon characters, including Thomas the Tank Engine and Dora the Explorer. It felt like I was a child again.

The procedures were extremely painful. A team of nurses and doctors held me in position and kept reminding me to breathe. The first camera went down my throat and wind pipe, and I wanted to gag. How they expected me to stay still I don't know. The second camera was inserted in my bottom and at first, all I could feel was the sensation of air being pumped, but each time the pain intensified. It was the most painful procedure I had ever experienced. I just wanted it to be over.

When it was finally over, I discovered that I would have to undergo more procedures. The doctor said that they couldn't complete the colonoscopy. 'There was an inflammation too big, so the camera couldn't go all the way through. We have taken a biopsy, and you will now be put in for an emergency CT scan. The biopsy result together with the scan result will determine what you have. You either have Crohn's disease or cancer.'

This was the first I had heard of the possibility of the 'C' word: cancer. 'You either have Crohn's disease or cancer' were words that played on loop in my mind for the next five days.

I was now 'hoping for the best but expecting the worst', the lyrics from Alphaville's 'Forever Young' bringing me some kind of bittersweet comfort. I'd fall asleep listening to that song on repeat. I googled Crohn's to learn it was a nasty disease; my best-case scenario.

I went through five days of not knowing what hand life had dealt me.

On 11th December 2014, a Thursday morning, I waited for a nurse to call me in. My appointment was moved from 10am to 9am. It was a crowded clinic and the waiting was exhausting, but once I was called in at 11am, the waiting didn't matter anymore. It was, in fact, a doctor who called me in, with the nurse alongside.

The doctor wasn't sure how much I knew, so he asked what I had been told five days earlier. Word for word I repeated: 'There was an inflammation too big, so the camera couldn't go all the way through. A biopsy was taken, and together with the emergency CT scan, the results will determine whether I have either Crohn's disease or cancer.'

He gently nodded his head, and quietly said: 'Yes, it's cancer.'

Time almost stood still. So many thoughts went through my mind. I silently affirmed to stay strong; strong for the doctor who had just broken the news, strong for the nurse who was sitting opposite, strong for my sister who was with me. Strong for my mum who was anxiously waiting at home for an update. Strong, even though all I wanted to do was break down, crumble and wash away into the ocean.

Maintaining my focus, I took out a pad of paper and began to take notes. I asked questions, and took in a lot of information. I strangely thought, 'I can do this', not yet fully knowing what was in store. I had an epiphany. My decade-long quest for personal and spiritual development was somehow preparing me for the biggest challenge of my life.

As the consultation came to a close, I had many more questions that could only be answered once a meeting with the oncology team took place. Yet, as I left the hospital, I could no longer hold back the tears.

I didn't have any words to say, I didn't know what to say. We just aimlessly walked up the high street. We went into a couple of stores; I think I was trying to maintain some regularity in what was to be the clichéd 'my life changes forever' moment.

And overnight my life was to change.

What was only meant to be a week off was now indefinite time off: my GP had signed me off for the long term. The projects I was working on became someone else's projects.

The future looked bleak. I was approaching my 32nd birthday on 20th December. The festive celebrations were around the corner, New Year was on its way, yet I wasn't sure if I would live to see another year. There was not much to be 'happy' about.

I cautiously broke the news to friends and family. I tried to protect them by saying, 'I have some tough news', or 'I have some shocking news', and then proceed to deliver the bad news. Whenever I talked about my condition, I couldn't quite hold my composure. Tears would come, my voice would tremble and tissues would be handed out to wipe my tears and clear my nose. Some people I bumped into in the streets. Some people I called randomly. To some people, I sent a message. I didn't know what I wanted to happen with each interaction. There was the heavy pain of the news inside me, and I thought that sharing the news with those closest to me would help ease the load. Each response was different. Some people had instant tears, some gave me a hug, some were speechless and some had questions. Sharing the news provided some sort of relief. A sense of 'I don't need to be alone; I don't need to do this on my own.'

## REFLECTION

Looking back to the moment I was diagnosed, I chose to stay strong to absorb as much information as possible. Even though I wanted to break down, I knew I would have time to cry afterwards, and I did cry as often as I felt the need.

It was a massive shock and I didn't know how things would pan out, but I chose to be open with my friends and family. I chose not to do what was ahead of me alone.

# CHOICE THREE

# TO ASK QUESTIONS

The impact from the diagnosis brewed inside me; my system was shocked to the core. My dad died of bowel cancer in his forties, when I was only two, and this suggested a genetic component in my disease. The C word, fuelled with uncertainty, got me thinking about death. There isn't a day that goes by since the diagnosis when I haven't thought about death.

With death staring me in the face, I had two primary questions:

First, '*What does this mean?*'

I remembered Viktor Frankl in the book Man's Search For Meaning, and his incredible story of concentration camp survival. I wanted to know what this diagnosis meant in the bigger scheme of things for me. I decided to begin my very own search for meaning.

Second, *'Do I choose to stay?'*

In the summer of 2012, I went to see Gabby B give a lecture in London. I remember in particular a question being asked by a member of the audience at the end of the talk. A woman asked why her mother had died from cancer. They had gone to see a famous spiritual healer who was said to have helped many people get better from life-threatening illnesses. Yet it didn't work for her mother. Gabby B asked if her mother had wanted to go, and whether she had chosen to go. The daughter instantly acknowledged that her mum had had enough of the pain and didn't want to suffer anymore. For some reason that idea stayed with me, it intrigued me, and two and a half years later I had that exchange at the forefront of my mind. The idea that no doctor or spiritual person can save a person if they decide that they no longer want to live resonated with me. I pondered the concept of a person's will to live, their choice in wanting to stay alive and to continue to breathe. There was a reason that conversation stayed with me. I found myself asking this pressing question.

I went to see my friend, mentor and integrative physician Dr Kim with those two key questions. An integrative physician is someone who treats a person's whole being. In addition to the physical symptoms, the physician works on various psychological, emotional and spiritual challenges one faces. I was in tears as I tried to articulate these questions. This wasn't an 'everyday conversation' and one that I certainly couldn't have had with everyone. Dr Kim instantly knew what I was asking. If I chose to stay, it would mean going deep into the abyss of my inner being. He said he would support me and walk side by side with me every step of the way, whatever I chose. I left Dr Kim with a sense of hope and a feeling that I would find meaning.

There were still several unanswered questions concerning my treatment and I waited a week, until I met my oncologist, to get these answers. Truth be told, I didn't know what an oncologist was. Google kindly helped me out: someone who dedicates their life to understanding and treating cancer.

Thanks to Google I also had two questions for the cancer specialist: What was the stage of the cancer? And what was the grade?

Stage 1 is the earliest; stage 4 the last. Stage 1 offers a better prognosis and a higher chance of survival, while stage 4 indicates a spread of the disease. The grade determines how fast the tumour is growing.

When the oncologist said my cancer was stage 4, and that I had 'a small chance of success', I was devastated. The grade didn't even matter anymore. Any hope I had of getting better was over. The tumour was inoperable and they planned to begin chemotherapy a week later, on Christmas Eve.

Their plan was to give me six cycles of chemo – a 48-hour infusion every two weeks – over a three-month period. They would connect me to a bottle attached to a peripherally inserted central catheter (PICC) line in my arm and send me home afterwards. I would need to eat, sleep and walk with the bottle attached for the duration. The aim of the chemo was to shrink the cancer, and if it did shrink, I would be put forward for an operation. If it didn't, I would need to undergo six months of chemo.

The news couldn't have been any worse. Hearing my chances were small, I questioned the point of having chemo. Yet, somehow, with my hands shaking, I managed to sign the consent form.

My shattered self continued to shatter, again and again.

It was dark, it was raining and it was miserably cold as I once again went to see Dr Kim. Once more, I poured my heart out. I was scared. I was an emotional wreck as I repeated the oncologist's blows.

'Mo, you are more powerful than the words of any doctor. The doctor is giving his opinion based on statistics. Whether you choose to stay or go, I am with you every step, with every decision. I will help you find your meaning,' he said.

Dr Kim's words were soothing and they brought me back to my centre. He reminded me of my two questions from a week ago. I knew the challenge ahead was real. It was serious. I couldn't just flow through this as I might have done with previous challenges. I knew I needed to dig deep within, and be prepared to go to places I didn't yet know existed.

It was in that moment, while lying back on the bed, hearing Dr Kim say that whatever I chose was okay, that I affirmed to choose to stay.

The next day I expressed my reservations about chemo to my GP, who said that I shouldn't lose hope. It looked like his eyes were welling up when he said he would have an open door for me, and that I could go and see him or call him at any time. He also said he wanted to see me regularly. The level of empathy shown was comforting.

As the days went by, I was angry, scared and upset. I knew the cancer was more serious than I had originally thought; that it wasn't going to be 'a walk in the park'. The enormity of the situation was sinking in; it felt surreal, not like anything I had encountered before. I began making peace with people, asking for forgiveness, and asking for prayers.

My 'small chance' was in contrast to the words from Dr Kim that my mind was more powerful than the words of any doctor. I remembered how I was in Dr Kim's clinic six months earlier asking for help with my identity crisis. Back then we did an exercise to create a vision for my life of no regrets; it was 'my picture'. That picture seemed like a distant memory, but Dr Kim reminded me of it and said it was vital now, more than ever.

## REFLECTION

From my personal development work, I was aware that the questions I asked would direct my focus.

I chose to search for meaning, and I chose to stay. Thanks to Dr Kim and to some soul searching, I chose to follow the belief that 'I am more powerful than the words of any doctor'. I chose to believe that the human mind is incredibly powerful. Ultimately, I chose to take responsibility for my health.

CHOICE FOUR

# TO BE ACTIVE

A specialist diagnoses the cancer, prescribes the course of action (chemo in my case), and then the patient goes home and lives with the consequences. So much of this approach felt wrong to me. My life changed in the seconds, minutes and hours that followed the diagnosis. My days and weeks were about to become unimaginably different.

Previously on a Sunday evening, I would be thinking about getting ready for a Monday morning commute, and mentally prepare myself for any drama awaiting me at work. I would wake up at 6am, have a shave and shower, make the hour-and-a-half commute and then work with my colleagues on projects that made a difference to the lives of students. Work was no longer an option as, physically, I couldn't make it in, and working remotely was a struggle as I found it difficult to focus. My employers left it to me to decide how involved I wanted to be.

Now I was questioning whether I'd be able to get any sleep, and if I did whether I'd wake up. My life revolved around a small perimeter of home and hospital.

I knew my interactions with people could dwindle as I didn't have the energy to go out, and with a weak immune system I didn't want to expose myself to germs and infections.

Hearing the prognosis was, on one level, devastating, but on another it was important. It gave me a barometer for my condition. I knew in no uncertain terms that the road ahead was going to be extremely tough. The oncologist's opinion on its own may have taken me on a different trajectory altogether, but following the conversation with Dr Kim, I was able to see a bigger picture. I was able to appreciate my role in what was about to happen. Instead of being passive and letting fate take its course, I decided to be active.

I set my intention to choose to stay. I chose to do what I could that was within my control. I chose an integrative approach to my cancer care.

Yes, I consented to the chemo, but I believed I would need more than chemo to deal with the psychological, emotional and spiritual challenges.

On a practical level, I knew my energy levels were about to be tested. I knew I was no longer as independent as I was accustomed to being since a young age. Reluctantly, I decided to accept help – help with my shopping, help with my travel, help with my cleaning, and help in many other ways of which I wasn't yet aware. This was not easy for me, and led to some heated exchanges. Seeing family members move my belongings as they rearranged my room was painful. They were setting things up so that I could go to sleep with a chemo bottle attached to me. Even thinking back to the chemo makes me feel nauseous.

I quickly realised that I needed to focus my energy on creating an environment of 'goodness'.

## MY RECORDS

As they were at the centre of my health care, I bought a folder to collect and monitor all my medical records. After each hospital appointment my file would get bigger. I asked for copies of scan reports, pathology reports and blood tests, and put them together with clinic notes as they arrived through the post. I kept a timeline of my appointments, the medication prescribed and a summary of what different doctors told me. I thought that having my own file would allow me to track my progress and that it might come in handy one day.

My dad left no medical records behind other than one letter from his surgeon confirming that he had transverse colon surgery for cancer. I wanted to make sure all my documents were in good order in case my nephews one day might want to learn more about my condition.

## MINDSET: BACK TO SCHOOL

I decided to learn as much as possible about my disease. I took down some old books from the shelf, wiped away the dust and began reading. I also bought new books about diet and nutrition, meditation, and cancer. I downloaded medical journals, and I began learning about cutting-edge science and technology – from epigenetics, quantum physics and neuroscience, to understanding the basics of biology and re-learning the mechanics of the human cell. I wanted to see if I could aid my healing through intention. A part of me also wished I had paid more attention in my biology lessons at school.

## NUTRITION AND DIET

Chemotherapy is commonly known to kill rapidly dividing cancer cells. In practice, this results in killing both good and bad cells, which weakens the body. Naturally, this would take its toll on me so I began taking nutrients and vitamins as part of my daily routine. I began experimenting with green juice recipes. 'Dr ABC' was a concoction of apples, beetroot and carrots. One juicer wasn't enough for me, so I bought a second. I would blend kale and spinach in one and add that to the mixture of cucumber, broccoli and anything else that was green in the other. I began taking shots of wheatgrass, but then one morning my body said 'no'. I had no choice but to spit it out as the taste was unbearable. Instead, I added wheatgrass to the juice. I removed meat from my diet and added plenty more vegetables. I did my best to eat as 'cleanly' as possible, although eating was sometimes a challenge, as the side effects from the chemotherapy included mouth ulcers and a loss of taste. I also had to keep an eye on my weight as I continued to shed kilos.

## MIND, BODY AND SOUL

In addition to my physical demands, my thoughts and feelings were being stirred. I made weekly or forthrightly visits to Dr Kim for help, and when I was unable, physically, to get to his clinic, we would speak via Skype. I will discuss how these sessions unfolded in later chapters, but, in a nutshell, they allowed me to explore my ever-evolving fears as I progressed with my treatment, and to revisit my wounds from the past to fully release my emotions. These sessions also enabled me to re-focus my mind, reminding me of my bigger picture and my quest for meaning.

## A NEW ROUTINE

With my regular routine disrupted, I knew I needed to create a new set of rituals. My mornings now included a variation of meditations, writing gratitude lists, gentle movements and listening to healing sounds. When possible I'd go for short walks. During the day I would listen to recordings of interviews with health specialists and motivational talks, in between reading and studying. I also found a reason to start writing posts for my blog, which I had stopped updating several years ago. Writing was a passion of mine, and blogging about my cancer allowed me to regain a connection with an old pastime, which in itself was therapeutic. Lots of people wanted to be kept up to date, and blogging allowed me to do this without having to message everyone individually.

## MEETING FRIENDS

It was easy to become isolated, my life revolved around hospital visits, treatment and recovering at home. Going out for social activities was not practical; the chances of catching infections were high, especially during the long winter. Yet, I was blessed to have friends who kept in touch. I would make arrangements to meet with different friends during my recovery week. These catch-ups allowed me to temporarily forget my health situation as I heard about the trials and tribulations of everyday life. These meet ups in local cafes gave me a reason to leave my enclosure and escape the world of cancer. I am grateful for these moments that continue to this day.

## REFLECTION

I chose to take control of my health and find ways of carving out some kind of new routine. I chose to stay in touch with friends whenever health allowed. I chose to share my journey with anyone interested through social media. I chose to 'take each day as it comes', and this became a new mantra for me; one that helped me through some very dark days.

# TO LIVE EACH DAY
## (EVEN THE BAD ONES)

I did my best to create a daily routine, but some days were difficult. There were times when I found myself lying idle on the sofa. There was always some form of sport playing on the television in the background, but on those days I'd have no energy to change the TV channel. I would have no appetite for food or my green juices. My mother would bring me plate after plate, glass after glass, along with my supplements. I would look at them despairingly and then turn away. All I wanted to do was sleep.

Sometimes I felt nauseous. Keeping sick bags to hand was crucial, but occasionally I didn't reach for them in time and created a mess. Each time I regurgitated, it felt like my insides were about to come out.

Chemotherapy was brutal. It took its toll on me.

I would go to the hospital on a Wednesday afternoon for blood tests, a weight check and a consultation with the oncologist to authorise the chemo. I would then see the pharmacist, who would prescribe medication to help with the side effects – tablets aimed at minimising the sickness and diarrhoea, and steroids to give me a boost. The entire process took hours. I was just one soul out of hundreds, perhaps thousands, waiting patiently in a hospital dedicated to cancer patients.

Seeing doctor after doctor walk along the corridor to pick up a file and call out a name filled me with dread because I wasn't sure what bad news they would have for me. Yet, a part of me hoped that it was my folder, just to get the clinic out of the way. Once my name was called out, the appointments were rather short: a checklist going through my experience from the previous cycle and a look at my blood test results, which would usually indicate that the chemo should be administered the next day.

The chemo days began early. These were the days I wanted to be over in a hurry, but they lasted the longest. There was a lot of waiting around. The day would begin with a nurse changing the PICC line dressing, followed by the first of several observations or 'obs' as the nurses called it, which involved checking my temperature, blood pressure and pulse. When all these were given the okay, there was a wait for the chemo to be ready.

Depending on how busy the chemo floor was, I'd either have a chair or a bed to lie on for the infusion. The nurses would give me various anti-sickness drugs, followed by two chemo infusions. The first infusion, if everything ran smoothly, would take almost two hours. After this, the nurses would connect me to the pump with the second infusion and prepare me to go home for at least 48 hours.

Being connected to the pump limited what I could do at home, so I would be eager to go back to the chemo floor on a Sunday morning, once every drop of chemo was inside me, to have the bottle disconnected.

This pattern continued for twelve weeks, for my first six cycles of chemo. Each cycle got more intense and the impact on my body was telling. I felt dirty as soon as the drops began entering my body.

Fatigue swept over me and doing simple daily actions, such as shaving, showering or even changing my clothes, felt like an achievement. I soon gave up on shaving and decided to see what I'd look like with a beard. 'Caveman' was the word I used to describe how I felt, until my barber, Chopper, shaped it for me and made me look tidy once more.

My hair didn't fall out, to the surprise of lots of people. Shortly after my first cycle, a relative called my mum to ask whether my hair had fallen out. It was also one of the first questions many people asked after hearing about my diagnosis, which was nonsensical to me. Hair was the last thing on my mind, yet was one of the first for others. Every time I went for a hair trim, Chopper and I would joke about how long we could go with the hair still there, although the thought of chunks of hair falling out as he washed my hair was a bit unnerving.

While my hair stayed, my weight dropped considerably, as did the haemoglobin levels in my blood. One afternoon, a doctor, while going through my pre-chemo checklist, casually dropped in that they had booked me in for a blood transfusion. Hearing those words freaked me out. Blood what? From my limited knowledge of medical terminology, this did not sound good at all. It turned out that my blood levels were too weak for chemo, and I'd need to be given blood to bring my levels back up, strong enough to handle the chemo. This was routine practice for the medics, but for me it was terrifying. I explained to the doctor that the way they say things can have a huge impact, and what might seem simple to them can sound daunting to a patient.

After I had my sixth cycle in March 2015, it was time for the CT scan. Memories from the first CT were still fresh in my mind as I went in. Lying on the bed, there is nothing you can do. The procedure takes just seconds, as the bed moves you in and out of the machine, but the results of those few seconds are crucial in determining the next steps. I prayed for a miracle.

I came home that afternoon and was getting ready to lie down on my couch when I received a call from an unknown number, which happened to be a doctor from the hospital. They had detected a blood clot in my lungs and wanted me to go into A&E within the hour. Once more I was resigned and I was petrified. Again, from my limited medical knowledge, I knew a blood clot was serious and the fact they wanted me back in immediately added to the anxiety.

It was a short trip to the hospital, but the evening proved to be rather long. My temperature rose, so I was monitored continuously. When the on-call oncologist came to see me, he said I would need blood thinning injections every day for six months, which didn't feel comforting at all. The fact that I would need to administer them myself made the idea less appealing. The doctor also said I would need to stay overnight for monitoring.

The room I was in was freezing cold, and the blankets they gave me didn't seem to make any difference. I fell in and out of sleep, while they attached me to a drip and carried on with their obs. It was during the early hours of the morning, at around 2am, that they found me a bed on a ward and wheeled me out of A&E. My family stayed with me until I reached the acute diseases ward. Once there, I fell in and out of sleep as another patient regularly screamed in agony. I later found out that he was suffering from a hernia.

In the morning, the doctors did their morning round. They said that I showed signs of an infection, but they couldn't detect where so they would need to do further blood cultures, which could take days to come back. They also said my oncology team would be around later to give me an update on my scan results.

The oncology team, in fact, came over the following day, and delivered some much-needed good news. They said my tumour had shrunk, and that they would now be handing me over to the surgical team for an operation. Hearing this news filled me with relief, gratitude and tears. In the first three months of challenging days, I had finally received some positive news.

I stayed in hospital for over a week, during which time I had a second blood transfusion, a few saline drips, and the suspected infection eventually left my body. It felt so good to be back home in my own bed.

## REFLECTION

Going through cancer involves facing a lot of bad news. Sometimes this news caught me off guard. Each time, I acknowledged the scare and the fear, and chose to surrender. The mantra 'this too shall pass' often came to my mind as I chose to hang in there, and endure another day.

# CHOICE SIX

# THE LITTLE THINGS

Going to bed each night was not easy. I was never sure if I would fall asleep, and, if I did, wake up in the morning.

In the darkest hours of some nights, I would wake up with severe abdominal pain. I'd pace around my room, yet find no relief. I'd sit on the toilet seat, again no relief. This would often happen. One night in desperation I fell to my knees, bedside, with my face drowning in the duvet. I began pleading with the pain. 'What do you want? What do you want me to do?' In that moment I felt a deep connection with life. I felt comfort, I felt relief. I was enveloped with love.

I would feel a connection to nature, to the universe, and would begin to appreciate the mysteries of life and the life force that was still alive within me. That same life force that keeps the planets in orbit; that takes an acorn and transforms it into an oak tree, or the caterpillar to a butterfly; that force that takes an embryo and breathes life into a baby. That life force was still inside me.

When I woke up in the morning, I'd always say thank you. Thank you for being alive. Thank you for being able to draw open the curtains. I would sit silently, close my eyes, breathing in air while feeling my lungs fill up. I'd begin to appreciate the amazing human body, the various systems at play in the body, helping a person function, helping me to function. The intricacy is fascinating, from the nervous system, to the respiratory, circulatory, reproductive, digestive, skeletal and muscular systems – the fact that each system is unique and intricate, yet works collaboratively in unison with the whole body, the whole person. It felt like a universe within me, so much within to explore. I began to thank my cells, my tissues, my organs, my body and all the systems I didn't know about for serving me all these years. I'd open my eyes with a sense of peace and gratitude.

I began appreciating the simple things I had previously taken for granted – little things, like being able to step out of my home, whether it was for an appointment or just for a breath of fresh air. Being able to stretch my arms out and feel the drops of rain on my palms, being able to see the sky change colour and feeling the wind blow against me. On the rare days I could walk to the shops and fill my own shopping trolley, I would have an extra spring in my step, an added smile.

I would think about conversations I had with strangers, from shop assistants to taxi drivers. I'd appreciate people going about their lives, with their own sets of challenges and dreams. I noticed the fast-paced world around me, yet I was content to move in slow motion. I'd think back over all the little things that made me angry and upset me. All the occasions I worked in my own time – a memory of replying to emails at 4am came to my mind. All those hours chasing buses and trains, and those stuck in traffic. I wonder how many of those hours were spent complaining about stuff that would now have little to no significance in my life.

I was now determined to create moments to remember.

My conversations with friends became deeper, more meaningful, they felt more special. Some friendships became stronger and I made new ones. My neighbour Jack was one of the first to learn of my cancer. I was going to visit my GP after being diagnosed when I bumped into him and shared the devastating news. Previously, conversations with Jack took place on the communal stairwell or on the street. Now I was having regular catch-ups with him over a cup of tea and a green juice. We took turns to visit each other, and learned more about each other in the space of weeks than we had in three decades. I'm sure between us we have theoretically solved the world's problems in our chats.

It was catch-ups with friends in person, over a phone call, or through an exchange of messages that helped me get through the tough days. The week in between chemos was my recovery week, and I'd always look forward to catching up with different friends.

I have five nephews and at diagnosis their ages ranged from between one and sixteen. They have always been a huge part of my life, and having a life-threatening disease meant uncertainty. I wasn't sure if I was going to see them grow up. I wanted to spend more time with them, when possible, being silly and finding any excuse to take a selfie. I would try to get them to support Tottenham Hotspur, my childhood football team, something I still carry on doing with varying success. They continue to make me laugh – and scream – at times, yet always make me marvel at their innocence and mischief.

I do my best when I'm with them to create moments and to capture them. I take them to the park and watch them play, or take them to the cinema. If my health allows, I take them to football matches. Hearing one of them say at his first live match, 'This feels like a dream' touched my heart and reinforced the power of little things.

Shortly after my diagnosis, one of them said, 'Mama (uncle), I've been practising how to give you a hug without hurting you' and proceeded to give me a delicate hug. Previously, we did 'super squeeze cuddles', but due to my 'tummy aches' he decided to modify the technique. These are moments I will always remember, moments that fill me with gratitude.

## REFLECTION

Choosing to appreciate life's simple moments is something that grounds me. Previously, I'd be living in the future, always planning a project of some sort, always being 'productive'. All of a sudden I was the project, and there was a lot less to do. This gave me an opportunity to just 'be', as much as possible. In the process, it allowed me to choose to connect deeply with friends and family, to deeply connect with life, and be okay with the concept of doing 'nothing'.

## CHOICE SEVEN

# TO EXAMINE MY LIFE

Getting accustomed to a new routine, surrendering to the bad days, and bad news, including the unexpected hospital stay, stretched me, but being grateful for all the little things helped me to navigate the days. Hearing the tumour had shrunk definitely brought a sense of relief, and was a sign that things were getting better, that the treatment was worth the pain.

Yet, being passed on to the surgical team wasn't getting me excited. I was terrified. The thought that they would cut open my abdomen and take out my insides filled me with dread. This was something else to bring to Dr Kim.

I had been visiting Dr Kim regularly now, for more than three months, and we had worked on my fears and revisited my old wounds. It was Socrates who said: 'The unexamined life is not worth living.' With death prevalent on my mind, it was my opportunity to examine my entire life and along the way, 'live a life worth living'. Working with Dr Kim enabled this examination.

## MY EARLY WOUND

When I was two, my dad died. I remember that day in 1985 when I was sitting under the dining table, pointing towards the sky saying, 'My dad is coming home on a plane.' I'd been making that gesture since the day he went to Bangladesh some six months earlier. That was my earliest recollection, waiting for my dad to come home, but that day I was told he would never be coming back. My mum, brother (9) and sister (7) were standing in front of me, tearfully shaking their heads in unison, saying, 'No, he won't be.' As a baby, I had no concept of death, yet that was an idea that I would begin grappling with. 'Surely they are teasing me, he must be coming back,' is what I remember thinking. During the days and weeks that followed, I still anticipated his return until one day I began to accept that he wouldn't be coming back. I would still point up towards the sky, repeating, 'My dad is coming home on a plane,' until one day I shook my head with my mum, who was in tears, and I repeated, 'He won't be coming back.'

I never got to know my dad, and I never asked about him. It was too painful to even mention him. All I knew was that he wasn't well and had gone to Bangladesh for herbal remedies and never returned home.

Later in life we would come to learn the truth. One afternoon in early 2013, I returned home to find my mum going through some old paper work. This included a suitcase belonging to my dad. There were so many folders and official looking documents. My mum gave me a couple of those to look at and asked me to confirm whether she was reading it right. My dad had undergone surgery for colon cancer in 1970, five years before he got married. He had hidden his illness from his family, and this was a huge shock to my mum. I took a photo of that letter, which was from his consultant, and thought that the information might come in handy one day.

As I connected the dots, I showed that photo to the doctor when I went in for my colonoscopy, and previously when I went to A&E. The letter no doubt helped to speed up my diagnosis. Coincidentally, when I mentioned the name of my dad's consultant to my oncologist, he said that the consultant had been one of his teachers. The world seemed a very small place.

I was now going through the same cancer, and was about to have the same operation. I was able to be closer to my dad than I ever imagined. I got to appreciate the pain he went through, and tried to understand why he had kept the condition a secret and travelled to Bangladesh.

## BANGLADESH

I went on my first trip to Bangladesh when I was five, in 1988. It was a short trip, and one necessitated through the illness of my grandma. I remember stepping out of Dhaka airport in the blazing heat. I instantly began sweating, and my arms turned red. There were thousands of people; I'd never experienced anything like that. The noise from the traffic, the heat, the vast number of people, it was too much. I screamed as beggars began reaching out to me, grabbing my hands. The street children mimicked my screams and laughed. My uncles came to collect us and wheeled our luggage to the car. The beggars reached into the car through the open window while we squeezed inside. My uncles handed out money in the hope that they would move on, but that only brought more to the car. The traffic was slow moving so we had to pull the windows up until we moved out of the city. It was my first experience of seeing poverty.

The village was different to the capital, Dhaka: fewer people, fresher air and more peaceful. One of my uncles took me for an evening walk and stopped by a stall on the side of the road. I chose a bread-like bun from what was available. As we walked back home I took a bite and had to spit it out. It tasted horrible and I couldn't bear to finish it. The guilt I felt was immense. I had seen so many kids with torn clothes, begging for money, and there I was wasting food. It was a moment that became a memory that would last forever.

The two weeks in Bangladesh went quickly. I saw my grandma in a lot of pain, with no control of her bowels or the ability to walk. The sight of adults carrying her to the bathroom for a wash, along with her screams of pain, are memories that have stayed with me. Shortly after coming back to the UK, we received news that my grandma had passed away.

In my short five years of learning about life and my place in it, I had experienced two deaths.

Then came the fear of losing my mum, and the fear of being an orphan. I'd seen orphans in Bangladesh, and felt an affinity with them, but I did not want to become one. It was a fear I could not speak about. I felt ashamed and embarrassed for having such thoughts. In primary school I loved PE, sports and play time, which helped me to forget the fear and pain. Yet, in the class room I would get lost in these thoughts as I became bored with class work. I would remember not having a dad and would worry about my mum and start to cry. The teachers would ask what was wrong, but I could never tell them the truth. I'd touch my tummy and say I had a tummy ache. I'd be sent to the school office, and Mrs World, the office lady, would call my mum. When mum came to collect me, it would bring a sense of relief and reassurance that she was okay. I was never able to tell her the real reason why I was upset.

Mum worked at several part time jobs, including childminding and sewing, while bringing up three kids, cooking, cleaning and taking care of the home. She did what she could to raise us, on her own, in a country away from her family with English as a second language. It was tough and I worried about her. A factory regularly delivered bags full of material requiring stitching – garments that would eventually be stocked in well-known shops. Mum would find time to put them through the industrial-type sewing machine, which had a huge foot pedal. As she put her foot down, the needle would start going up and down, making a drumming noise. This scared me, as I feared she would trap her fingers. As a toddler, I would try to stop her by emptying cupboards and drawers that I could reach. In my broken English I would say 'Amma machine nah'.

As I recalled each story to Dr Kim, I would be in tears. I was holding all this hurt inside. Dr Kim, at times, welled up too. He knew when to talk and when to stay silent. The process was cathartic, albeit emotional. Dr Kim observed how it was my tummy I'd point to in my pretence as a child to make sure my mum was safe, and now, in adulthood, it was my tummy that was really in pain and in need of surgery. There was something profound and meaningful in this connection.

## REFLECTION

Choosing to revisit wounds was difficult, but I realised I was carrying that energy inside me. It was stored as hurt, regret and suffering. Even though as an adult these emotions weren't things I thought about, they were, nonetheless, harboured in my consciousness. Choosing to open up and release the past was part of my emotional healing.

CHOICE EIGHT

# THE TRUTH
## (MAKING MY PRIVATE PUBLIC)

Revisiting my childhood wounds with Dr Kim was a long, overdue emotional release. Piecing together the imagined fears that shaped much of my childhood allowed me to see a bigger picture of my life, but there was still a lot left to explore.

Topics that I never thought possible to talk about were now being brought out into the open. I began telling my mum about the stories. Both of us shed tears as I recalled my memories of the sewing machine, the fake tummy pains and my fear of being an orphan.

Talking about these memories no doubt set some hurt free. I decided to talk about my cancer story to a wider audience through social media and began to make my blog posts public.

It was my opportunity to be as authentic as possible by writing about both the good days and the bad.

As I shared my inner thoughts, my fears and my hopes, the response was overwhelming. I remembered a time when I wanted to be 'inspiring', but in the midst of my cancer all I wanted was to be alive. Yet, people would send me messages saying that what I had written truly moved them and that it was inspiring. When I 'let go' of wanting to be a certain way, I was, ironically, being described as such.

One evening my mum opened up to me with a fear of her own as she told me a story.

*Once upon a time in the 1800s in East Bengal (now Bangladesh), a mother was sitting underneath a tree, weeping in desperation. By her side were two young children, her two sons. One sat on either side of her, blanketed around her arms. As night was falling and cold weather was about to set in, the mother feared how the dark hours would pass. Every day, she asked the same questions. What future could she give her sons, aged four and two? She wept as the thought of not providing them shelter for the night pained her. In addition, she couldn't provide food for them during the day. It was a struggle for her; it was a struggle for the boys. She lost hope. She began to cry hysterically.*

*Meanwhile, two men from a nearby village were walking home and crossed paths with her.*

*Upon hearing the sounds of desperation, the men stopped and discovered the woman sitting with her two boys.*

*They asked her what was wrong. The woman explained her situation. 'I can't give these children a future; I don't know what to do.'*

*The men had a conversation, and then turned to
the woman to make her an offer.*

*In their wisdom the men proposed to take her
two sons and give them a future that she could not
possibly imagine for them. In doing so, they would
take away her day-to-day struggles of bringing up
her children.*

Upon hearing this, I was stunned. I thought they would
offer to give the family some money or some form of shelter for the night. Their proposition was shocking; didn't
they think about the pain of separating a mother from
her children, and the children from their mother? Could
such pain even be described or felt by anyone else? Could
they not offer to look after them all? Could they not find
another way?

On reflection, the buying and selling of people, trag-
ically, was the norm. In the West, the transatlantic slave
trade was widely documented in history books, and I have
no doubt similar practices took place in the East.

*The mother, upon hearing the proposition cried
in desperation. Eventually, she said: 'I will give my
children to you, but on one condition. You need
to treat them as your own. You must ensure that
you bring them up as you would your own children: with love, with warmth, with heart. You must
cherish them.'*

*At the same time, she dropped a potential curse.
'If you treat them any other way, your family and*

*future generations will suffer. The pain that I, as a mother, will have to go through by letting my children go cannot be expressed. You treat them well, or your family lineage will be damned. Men will die young and the grass will continue to grow until no people remain. You have been warned: look after them as your very own.'*

*The men agreed to the woman's condition and took the children, leaving the mother and her heart crying to the ears of the universe.*

*The two men decided to take a child each. The boys were not only separated from their mother, they were separated from each other. Each boy went into a new home, with the promise of a new family.*

*One family did as the mother stipulated and looked after the child as their own. They schooled him, and fed him and gave him a decent upbringing.*

*The other family were to be cursed, just as the mother prophesied. They named the boy 'Ghulam', which means a 'servant of God' in Arabic. Only this child was to become a slave of the family. They disregarded the mother's wishes and so the spell was set.*

My mum went on to tell me that one of the men was my great-grandad from my dad's side of the family. My great-grandad had gone against the desperate mother's wishes. This was a lot to take in.

Could the curse be real? Men were dying young from generation to generation, just as the mother had warned. My grandad died as a young man. From what I understand,

my dad didn't really get to know his dad. My dad died rel-
atively young and my dad's brother died in his twenties.

Is this folklore, a myth, a legend? Was this history? If
the curse was true, would I be next?

What I know is that this story has been passed on from
generation to generation. The story has been passed down
to me. Whether I believed in a curse wasn't important.
What was important was the energy that this story carried.

I knew intuitively that I had to balance the energy with
love: to feel the mother's pain and heartache and to seek
forgiveness; to feel the children's pain and suffering and
seek forgiveness; to bring love to the surface, to collapse
the curse, to close the legend, to bring a mother and her
children together under the name of love. I wasn't sure
how I would do this though. This would be another area
to explore, if I made it past surgery.

## REFLECTION

Choosing to be as authentic as I possibly could was a conscious decision, but it was one which allowed me to just
'be'. I didn't want to pretend to make people feel a certain
way. I just wanted to express myself as honestly as possible. If I was angry or sad, or grateful and optimistic, I
wanted to be real. What I found was that the more real I
was, the more people were able to be honest back.

CHOICE NINE

# TO TRUST

One of the most dreaded days of my life had arrived. Over the past five months, I'd had cameras inserted in me, which resulted in a late stage cancer diagnosis. I'd been through six cycles of chemo, blood transfusions and a week-long stay in hospital after a blood clot was detected in my lungs. Now it was time for surgery.

A few days before the operation, Dr Kim arranged a meeting with his colleague Daljeet, because I was feeling apprehensive about the surgery. The plan, explained to me during the pre-assessment meeting at the hospital, was to cut me open and take out my colon and anything else they thought was necessary. The consent form included permission to take out the stomach, the abdominal wall and the spleen. 'What would be left of me?' I questioned.

Daljeet helped me to reconnect with my dreams and my sense of purpose. I recalled all my early ambitions: the dream of being an Olympic gold medallist and the dream of lifting the football World Cup. As a kid I pretended to be a news reporter. I would sit with a cardboard box cut out as a TV set, and I would proceed to read the nine o'clock news. As I became older, I became a truth seeker. I wanted to know the mysteries of the universe. I wanted to change the world. I wanted to do something about the poverty, the inequality and the suffering I saw. I wanted to work with orphans and street children; that affinity I felt as a five-year-old was still strong. I wanted to open a 'School of Hope', where kids would be allowed to explore their natural talents and pursue their passion. Connecting all the themes together, it was clear I wanted to play on a global stage, to share truth, to make a positive change in people's lives and, in the process, the world. This process allowed me to focus on the reasons to come through the other side of surgery to eventually fulfil my inner vision.

## THE DAY OF SURGERY

It was an early start and I had strict instructions to follow from the pre-assessment team. I had to stop eating the evening before and I was given a drink filled with electrolytes to take at 5am. This was to keep me hydrated. I took a shower and packed a bag in preparation for another hospital stay.

We got to the hospital at 6am and I was called in by the anaesthetists at just after 2pm.

In between the waiting I met my surgeon. This was the man who had broken the news of my cancer all those months ago. He ran through the plan and introduced me to a second surgeon, and mentioned that there would be a third in the operating theatre – a specialist for the stomach. I would also have the registrar, present when I went under the knife. Having four surgeons looking after me reassured me that I was in good hands, but it also underscored the seriousness of the procedure ahead.

I met the stoma nurses, who marked an X on the right-hand side of my belly, indicating the ideal spot for my new pouch to collect my stools. It felt surreal. A few months earlier I had no idea what an ostomy bag was. If everything went to plan I would be the owner of one later that day.

Several nurses and medics came to check my weight, temperature, height, blood pressure and pulse during the day. The paperwork was explained to me several times by different people, reiterating what was going to happen to me. I signed the consent form and once more wondered what body parts I would be left with.

During the wait, I was accompanied by my mum, sister and uncle. A number of messages were exchanged privately and on social media from friends wishing me the best. It was an emotional time, as I gave my mum a hug, telling her everything was going to be okay. Dressed in nothing but my green hospital gown and matching tights, I handed my phone to my sister and said goodbye as I was escorted by a nurse to the lift taking me closer to the operating theatre.

It was time for me to be put to sleep to go under the hands of the surgeons. The anaesthetists talked me through the procedure one final time. I wanted reassurance that I would not wake up in the middle of the operation. They assured me this wasn't possible and said there would be someone monitoring me. If anything like that showed the slightest hint of happening, they would increase the dosage. They helped me to relax and reminded me that there was no rush. I lay on my side as they found the right place to insert the first needle in the back.

That's all I remember, until I woke up in agony in the recovery theatre. A tube inserted through my nose and down my throat was making me gag, which I wasn't expecting. Despite all the explaining beforehand, they had left a crucial part out. I also felt a lot of pain in my upper chest. Nurses informed me that I would be taken to the intensive care unit (ICU). They said they would increase the pain relief and advised me to focus on my breathing. I could see that it was 6pm from the clock on the wall.

When I got to the ICU a number of family members were waiting to see me. I had no desire to speak and I didn't even want to know how the operation had gone or what body parts I had left. I had no sensation from the chest downwards. This meant I couldn't even push myself up the bed when I slid off the pillow.

I wasn't allowed any food and only allowed to take sips of water, which was difficult to do because of the nasogastric (NG) tube. I was attached to a catheter that collected my urine, along with my new stoma. A drip provided me with the necessary nutrients. I was given a pain relief pump and was advised to press it every few minutes to ease the pain.

While trying to take some sips of water, I vomited a green liquid and made a mess in the process. The quality of care I received exceeded all my expectations. I was cleaned without any fuss and was well looked after. I fell asleep, occasionally waking up to see the nurses on night watch. I can't remember what we talked about as I was too drugged up, but I remember feeling that I was in safe hands.

In the morning, my surgeon came to see me and said he was very happy with the operation and that 'they had taken out all the cancer'. They cut out my colon as expected, and only 'a wedge off my stomach', while the spleen and the abdominal wall were both left intact. Hearing the update was a huge relief and gave me hope that I was on my way to recovery.

I was soon taken to the regular ward where I met my stoma nurse, who taught me how to clean and change my bag. I met my physio team, who, day by day, retrained me to sit up on my own again, to stand, take steps and, eventually, to walk freely. The day came when the nurses were happy to take out the staples that were holding my open wound in place. The skin had fascinatingly meshed together to form a scar, allowing the staples to be tweezed out. I could hear a patient in the next bed screaming when he had his taken out, so I wasn't looking forward to my turn, but when the nurses began, I didn't feel terrible pain. As I became able to walk confidently again, my catheter was taken out. When the doctors were happy that my lungs were drained, the NG tube came out. I was eased back into eating food. Surprisingly, ice cream was what the doctor ordered for me. I had porridge for breakfast and soup for my other meals to begin with. As I got used to eating again, I was given regular food.

In total, I spent over two weeks at the hospital. The fear I had prior to the operation was balanced by the vision I held for the future. I went from being numb with very little sensation to re-learning how to be mobile. The doctors gave me the all-clear to go back home. I was trained to look after my stoma and advised not to do any heavy lifting for six weeks. I was to be handed back to the oncology team for my post-op chemo cycles.

## REFLECTION

Surgery was scary. Expressing my fears to Dr Kim gave me a release and a reconnection to my dreams. There was a lot of uncertainty in the build-up to surgery and afterwards. I trusted the process and surrendered while being unable to move. One patient on my ward said it took him months to relearn how to walk after he had had a similar operation. I chose to acknowledge the uncertainty, and, where possible, process the rational or irrational fear with the help of others.

## CHOICE TEN

# DESTINY

After I returned home after surgery, a month went by very quickly. Once more, I found myself in the presence of an oncologist at the cancer clinic. I wasn't looking forward to more chemo, and I let the doctor know that. He told me not to worry and that 'the worst was over', as he signed off the paper work to restart me on the chemo.

It was the same as before, with each cycle taking more than two days. I had another set of six in store, one every two weeks, over three months, which was to be followed by a scan. Once more, the side effects were brutal. I carried on with the rituals to get me through the good days and the bad, and I used the recovery week to catch up with friends. A carer came to help me once a day with domestic support and assisted me for my walks. The dizziness I was now experiencing put me at risk from having black outs and the assistance was most welcome. As the cycles came to an end, I could see that I was slowly going back to my regular life. Under the agreement of the doctor, my PICC line connected to my right arm was taken out. I began readying myself mentally.

It was now August 2015, and I ventured out of my health-enforced perimeter of hospital and the local cafés. I nervously attended a wedding in Birmingham, which was my first social occasion since I was diagnosed. I agreed with my employers to go back on a phased return. Initially, this was two days a week, with restricted hours to 'feel my way' back into work. Making the journey to Kingston was emotional. My organisation had made many changes, with a restructure and transitional arrangements still in progress. We had a new office, new staff starting and old staff leaving. We were also heading into a new academic year with induction activities being planned. There was a lot to catch up on, and I had a project to feel excited about. 'Change The World' workshops for new students starting university were sessions I had run for the first time a year earlier. They were on the schedule again this year and I was tasked to deliver them. University life provides students with several opportunities to explore their interests and passions, and I designed these sessions to connect students to what they enjoy doing and find a way to make a positive difference in the world at the same time.

After a month at work, I was ready to increase my days to three a week. I had familiarised myself with the new team, re-connected with former members of staff and was ready for a fresh start. Yet, there were other plans in store for me. I had an appointment scheduled with my oncologist to give me an update on the post-op chemo CT scan, which I'd had a month previously. As I hadn't heard anything from the hospital I assumed everything was okay. 'If anything was wrong they surely would have called?' was my thought process. On a previous occasion, they had called me the same day with the frightening blood clot news.

The doctor called my name, and I was nervous as I walked with him down the corridor and into his room. I was hoping for the word 'remission', and then to be handed back to the surgical team for a conversation about reversing my stoma. The consultation went differently to the script in my head.

'It's bad news, there is more cancer', more devastating news from the oncologist. I was stunned; this wasn't something I had anticipated hearing. The cancer had progressed right through the chemo into my lymph nodes. It seemed that the doctors weren't expecting these results either as there was no plan of action in place. He said he would check with colleagues at the Royal Marsden whether they had a new form of treatment called immunotherapy. Things were now 'up in the air'. Immunotherapy was something I had never heard of. He told me to come back the following week, and if the Marsden had this new treatment he would send me straight there. If not, I would need a different type of chemo.

It was life repeating itself once more. I was dejected, broken and resigned. The tears once more flowed as I walked up the high street quietly. This time, I had gone to the hospital on my own. Instead of being told I was in remission, I was told it was a relapse. Once more, I was to return home to deliver bad news to my mum. I didn't know how to say that there was more cancer, that I would need more treatment. The news was tough to take in. I was once more questioning life; why was this life, my life, so cruel?

A week later, I was informed that I would need a second line chemo as the Royal Marsden could not offer me immunotherapy. This more aggressive form of chemo was to be given indefinitely, but initially for six cycles in the same format as before.

Just when a sense of normality was returning in my life, it was about to get very uncertain again. More cancer, stopping work, new treatment: it was like I was starting the nightmare all over again with no concrete plan in place.

There was no way I would be able to continue with work, because there was no timetable for any recovery. In consultation with my employers, we decided to call my time at Kingston to a close.

By now I'd learned that with cancer, things change very quickly. I instantly started to hand back my work, and braced myself for more chemo. I had one final piece of work left to do, which was to deliver the last 'Change the World' session. It coincided with a chemo cycle. Plugged into the bottle, and escorted by my nephew on my journey, I made one final trip to work. Delivering the session to a packed room of enthusiastic students showing empathy and passion for the challenges they saw in the world was heartening. The topics they discussed, with the desire to do something, made my final day gratifying. It was a shame I couldn't be part of their future. I packed up my last remaining belongings from my desk and said goodbye to my colleagues.

I struggled through each chemo cycle, somewhat going through the motions as best as possible. Each cycle seemed to arrive too quickly. I was sick to the core. Wanting to get a sense of the plan ahead, I probed the doctors. One of them broke me with the words 'disease management'. He said surgery was not an option, and chemo would be offered to me for the foreseeable future – another six cycles after the scan. It was very unlikely the cancer would go away; at best the chemo would keep it under control.

Living the rest of my life on chemo was not the destiny I wanted.

## REFLECTION

This phase of the cancer story was very different from before. Earlier, there had been a plan in place with light at the end of the tunnel. I was not expecting the curveball. One of my mentors described it as the corner, which I thought I had turned, being stretched a bit further. This time, everything was 'up in the air', as an oncologist described it, while another mentioned 'disease management'. All I could do was choose to trust, and this time choose destiny. Surely destiny would find me a way.

CHOICE ELEVEN

# THE UNKNOWN

My one-year cancer anniversary had arrived: 11th December – a day I never thought I'd see, yet a day that will forever be a milestone. Every day during the year has mattered and continues to do so; every day is filled with the unknown. In the space of a year, I'd had eighteen gruelling cycles of chemotherapy, together with all the side effects, the blood transfusions and the blood clot. I'd had a major operation, gone back to work, only needing to quit all too soon. Learning to live life differently, I had to take one day at a time. At best, I could only think ahead as far as the next scan.

Yet the next scan brought further bad news, three doses' worth.

*'The chemo's not working.'*
*'The cancer is growing.'*
*'There's no more treatment available.'*

Three pieces of information that technically meant my cancer was terminal. On one level I got my wish, no more chemo, but on another level there was no other option. I remained beyond calm; I remained focused. 'What can we do?' I asked.

I quizzed the oncologist about immunotherapy, something he had asked the Royal Marsden about in September. He told me that because my cancer had a genetic component, which they confirmed following a lengthy genetics test, I was a very good candidate. I have something called Lynch Syndrome, passed on from my dad. Immunotherapy was still in the research stages for my cancer, but the studies had shown an incredible response rate for Lynch Syndrome cancers. The only problem was immunotherapy was not available on the NHS. When I asked how much the drug cost, I was told I needed to be 'a millionaire'.

The oncologist said he would put in an application to the NHS for an individual treatment request, but warned it could take months to hear back. He said he would forward me to a research institute to find me an immunotherapy clinical trial. Terminal didn't quite mean terminal just yet. It wasn't over for me.

As the end of the year approached and I turned 33. My nephew Ejaz, who was to turn six the next day, called me to sing 'Happy Birthday'. He began counting the years from one to 33, and then carried on counting after thirty three. We both laughed and I thought to myself, I'd happily take those extra years.

New Year 2016 began with more unknowns.

I was looking forward to going to my first football match for a long time. My friend Dave, who I met back at the students' union, was now living in Dubai. He was coming to London and had booked tickets for Tottenham vs Leicester City. Our respective teams were miraculously challenging for the title. As we arrived at the stadium, we enjoyed catching up. Dave was on the cusp of completing a world record – travelling to every single country in the quickest time – and hearing stories from his adventures was inspiring. Yet, as we took our seats for the match, it was to become a horrible experience. My stoma leaked, creating a mess. I didn't have spare supplies as I avoided taking a bag upon stadium security advice. The shit, quite literally, hit the fan. Dave assured me that he couldn't smell anything, so we stayed the entire game. Tottenham ended up losing the game and Leicester went on to win the league. When I got home that night, it took a couple of hours to get cleaned up with my mum's help. It was an episode to be forgotten as soon as possible.

The research institute eventually met with me in mid-January and informed me that the immunotherapy they anticipated had been delayed. They were, however, able to offer me a phase 1 study: a drug being administered to patients for the first time. For a drug to be approved, it needs to go through four phases, and then go through a cost analysis process to see if it is worth making available on the NHS. This entire process can take over a decade. While we waited for immunotherapy, the doctors thought this new trial was worth a try. I was going to be the twenty-third patient in the UK.

Two months into the trial, I was given more bad news. The doctor overseeing my care called to inform me that the tumours were getting bigger and showing signs of spreading into other areas. I was taken off the trial immediately. The situation was very bleak, and time was running out for me. The immunotherapy trial wasn't going to start anytime soon, and the one that was opening up would not accept me as it was only taking patients who had not had any previous treatment. My oncology team persisted in trying to get me treatment by completing applications to different drug companies, asking if they would provide the medication on compassionate use, but these applications were rejected.

Almost four agonising months passed, and getting an answer from the NHS was of paramount importance. I had been in touch with my nurse every month, checking in to see if they had received an answer. Every time the answer was, 'We haven't heard anything'. I was finally called in for a clinic appointment to get an update.

I was at the hospital, watching a cricket match on my phone, while waiting to be called in. Bangladesh was playing India in the T20 World Cup and was on the verge of an incredible victory when a doctor called for me. Quickly turning the phone off, my attention moved to the doctor who wasted no time in telling me the decision. The NHS had declined to pay for the treatment.

I was lost for words. Waiting all those months to hear a 'No' was tough. All my options had run out. Ultimately, the drug cost too much.

Meanwhile, there was a lump visible on my neck, which the doctors were certain was cancerous. They said I would need radiation for it. I asked whether they would be able to radiate the other tumours at the same time. The doctor explained that radiation burns the tumour, and the sites of the others were too close to organs, which would also burn in the process.

I asked whether I'd be allowed to travel to Makkah, in Saudi Arabia for a week-long mini pilgrimage, which had been planned two months earlier. He said that would be fine, and in fact a change in environment would do me good.

Straight after the appointment, Ru arranged to meet with me. I'd known Ru since I was a kid, when we'd lose the concept of time while playing football at Regents Park. I remember we'd start playing in the afternoon, and would only think about stopping and going home when it turned dark. When Ru heard I had cancer, he called me immediately and said, 'Mo, I don't know anything about cancer, but I'm here for you.' He continued to stay in touch, organising social gatherings to get me out of the house. Growing frustrated at the lack of treatment, he wanted to help. When I gave Ru the latest update from the hospital, he suggested a fundraising campaign for the treatment.

'Let's fundraise,' he said. 'Let's do something.' I was not in a place to do that. I said I'd be happy to raise money for a cause, for the 'School of Hope' that was in my vision. 'I don't care about your vision, I care about you. If we can keep you alive, your vision gets bigger.' Ru left me with lots to think about. He advised me to ask my imam what his thoughts were about fundraising, when I travelled to Makkah in the following days.

## REFLECTION

I described the previous phase as 'up in the air', but this phase was uncharted territory. I had chosen the unknown with a phase 1 trial, but it had yielded no benefit. I was now asked to think about choosing to fundraise – another unknown for me. The only certainty was that without treatment the cancers would continue to grow. I had a lot of soul-searching to do and had the perfect space to do it, at the holiest site in Islam.

# TO SEARCH

Back in December 2015, when I was coming home from my one-year scan, I bumped into my mum's friend on the bus. We had a short conversation as I was about to get off in a couple of stops, but in that time she asked if I had been to Saudi Arabia for an Umrah, a mini pilgrimage. I did, in fact, make this spiritual journey with my mum in 2006. I didn't think much of the conversation as I quickly reached my stop and walked home.

When I got home I answered the phone to hear the voice of Cha Cha, an uncle who lives in Saudi, who called to check up on us. Cha Cha had been our guide, taking us from site to site and helping us to perform the rituals, when we made the trip for Umrah.

Later that evening, my mum was watching TV when an advert came on promoting Umrah trips. She commented on the prices and I asked if she wanted to go. She looked at me with a resigned look, questioning who would take her. Unexpectedly, and even surprising myself, I said I would. She asked whether my health would allow me to make the journey, and I said I'd ask the doctors.

At the time, I didn't make a connection between those three events. It was only a month later in January, when my mum started to make calls about the possibility of the trip and found several packages that I reflected on those three separate encounters. They had spontaneously arrived together to bring about the possibility of my making a second trip. My doctors were happy for me to go, and we made plans to travel during the Easter Holidays in April. I spoke to an imam about one tour that interested me and booked it. I was looking for one which would allow me to take in the history while performing the rituals. My intention was to absorb as much history and meaning as possible.

The time had come to make the journey. It was the first time since I had been diagnosed that I was leaving the country. Before flying, I packed extra supplies for my stoma in various bags as I didn't want any messy leaks. I had medical letters about my condition in case they were needed, but thankfully the flights went ahead smoothly.

We began the trip in Medina, the city in which Prophet Mohammed (peace be upon him – pbuh) found refuge after being expelled from Makkah. When Mohammed (pbuh) began teaching Islam in the 7th century, the rulers felt threatened by the teachings and the vast number of people joining the religion. They wanted him to stop preaching and eventually sent death threats. Medina was the place Mohammed (pbuh) made home, and is a place

Muslims visit when performing the Umrah. It is a very peaceful place.

The Umrah follows in the footsteps of Mohammed (pbuh), marking the route he took when he finally returned to his birth home in Makkah. We visited all the historical sites and landmarks, including Mount Noor, the site where Mohammed (pbuh) would spend hours meditating. It was also the site where Angel Jibril (Gabriel) began revealing the Quran. We visited Mount Arafat, the place from which Mohammed (pbuh) delivered the famous Last Sermon. I learned that this was also the site in the Islamic teaching where Adam and Eve reunited after being sent down from heaven. Hearing the history and associated stories was fascinating and visiting the sites was emotional.

In Makkah, I performed the ritual of circling the Ka'aba seven times, wearing just two sheets of cloth – the exact same cloth that I will be buried in. It felt surreal, like I was preparing to die.

After one of my prayers finished in Makkah, I was looking at the Ka'aba, which was straight in front of me. There were so many people, male and female, from so many parts of the world. Different races and nationalities; some young, some old, some in good health, others not so, all there to surrender to God, wearing the simplest of clothing. I wondered whether I'd have another opportunity to come here.

My brother called to me to say a relative had just passed away. He had been suffering with cancer and his time had come. Upon hearing the news of someone dying, Muslims say, 'We belong to Allah, and to Him we shall return.'

There I was staring at the House of God, knowing that I too will one day pass.

After every single prayer, five times a day, in both Medina and Makkah, there was always a funeral prayer. It was a reminder that life is short.

Makkah was extremely busy and crowded. There was so much construction and development going on that it seemed very different from when I was there previously. The hotel we stayed in was in the incredible Clock Tower building, which had a mall full of shops and brands that were recognisable. The juxtaposition between the material and spiritual world was intriguing. Outside the hotel, you could turn one way and shop and dine to your heart's content, or turn the other way and spend time at the mosque enriching the soul.

I asked my imam Sheikh Madani whether he had time for me to interview him, as I had so many unanswered questions from the visits to the historic sites. Sheikh Madani, who studied in Medina for a number of years, kindly gave me time one evening. I raced through my questions, making notes as I went along. Questions clarifying time frames of when the Islamic calendar starts, how the Umrah began, why hair is either shaved or clipped at the end. As we closed off the interview, I told him that this Umrah felt like I was preparing to die, and he reinforced that that was indeed the purpose of the spiritual trip.

I had one final personal question to ask. 'Sheikh, the NHS have refused to pay for my treatment, my cancer is getting worse, my friend wants to fundraise, what shall I do?' He asked me a couple of questions about the condition and treatment, and said it was Prophet Mohammed's teaching to seek treatment, and so he advised that I had a 'duty to seek treatment'. If that meant fundraising, then that is what I needed to do. He vowed to give me his full support.

It was soon time to return home and leave the holy land behind, not knowing whether I'd ever come back. In London, I would have more soul-searching questions to answer.

## REFLECTION

I set out for Umrah with the intention of learning as much as possible, while fulfilling my religious obligations. I thought if I was going to die, this would be one last opportunity to give something back to my mum. I chose to ask my sheikh for his guidance, and was told I had a 'duty to seek treatment'. It was now a question of how I would fulfil that duty. Fundraising still didn't feel right and I was far from accepting that course of action.

CHOICE THIRTEEN

# HOPE

As I flew back from Saudi, I had a new-found duty to seek treatment. Fundraising, however, was the very last resort. I wanted to try everything possible before going down that route.

I did a search to find out who my local MP was, to see if they could help. Keir Starmer was one year into the role, having replaced the incumbent who'd been in place all my life. There happened to be a 'Meet Your MP' open session that evening. I decided to go with my uncle straight after my hospital appointment. The appointment was to find out more about the immunotherapy and to book radiotherapy for the lump in my neck. The referral to the radiation team was straightforward, but getting information about the drug was proving difficult. I learned that other patients had been denied the same drug, and that was the reason they had said they would not fund mine either. I still couldn't fathom why it had taken them four months to come back with that response.

Later that day, I met Keir and his advisor, and they took on my case immediately. Over the days and weeks that followed, it was clear that the political route would take a while. There were letters and phone calls back and forth between the hospital, the NHS and the Department for Health for months.

Regrettably, fundraising was becoming inevitable.

Before any fundraising could begin, I needed to get a grasp of how much I would need to raise. Finding the price was proving to be difficult and when given an estimate of £20,000 per month, over a one- to two-year period, the prospect was daunting. The maths was simple, yet the numbers were scary. I decided to look at options abroad and connected with doctors in the US and India. My friends and family also made enquiries, but whichever way we looked at it, it was going to be expensive and unrealistic.

I was nowhere near ready to go out and beg for my life. I questioned the price put on life and whether I was worthy to carry on living. Very quickly, I found myself in a depressive cycle. I would wake up, sit on the sofa and stare at the TV, not really watching what was on. I didn't shower or change my clothes for days, which felt like weeks. I cancelled appointments with friends and stopped carrying out all the rituals and routines that I had become accustomed to. The thought of having another green juice filled me with anger, and I said to myself, 'Fuck It, if I'm going to die, at least I'm going to enjoy my food.'

Relatives came to visit me. Some would put their hands on my head and around my face; some would give me a hug, while others would tell me to pray. I was in no mood to talk. I would watch my mum cry in front of me. I almost felt I was done, I'd had enough.

And then one Friday afternoon, I had an appointment with Roberta from my students' union days. Roberta was over in London from Brazil for a short stay, and we had arranged to have a catch-up. Sitting on my spot on the sofa, my internal dialogue went something like: 'I can't cancel on Roberta, I don't know if I'll ever see her again.' With that thought, I got ready and went out to meet her.

We met in one of my favourite cafes, Yumchaa, which always had a good selection of carrot cake. It felt good to come out, get some fresh air and connect with an old friend. Roberta said her husband Philipe would join us later, and so when someone came from behind covering my eyes with their hands and said 'Hello,' I was startled. I was expecting Philipe, but this sounded like someone totally different, someone with a Brummie accent. 'No freaking way!' It was Dave, who had flown over from Dubai and had taken a detour via London before heading up north. He made the trip to join us, which overwhelmed me. The three of us from the students' union days were together again. This had only happened twice in the last decade. I had no idea that they had planned this meet up. Dave, who I last saw at that forgetful football match, the same Dave, who some ten years earlier told me that if I resigned from the SU, I'd be running away my entire life. This special moment began to shift things for me. I was surprised, I was grateful. I re-connected with all the little things once more.

The following day, Ali, my former personal trainer took me for lunch, and I ordered a pizza. Not something I would have done in front of Ali back in my training days. We reminisced about how much progress I had made during those days until a shoulder injury took me out. As we finished catching up, Ali asked whether I'd like to step into my old gym to see the changes. The last time I went in was a sad day, towards the end of 2014, and that was to cancel my membership. As I went inside, the music was loud, playing Pompeii by Bastille, one of my favourite bands. The gym had a new layout, new machines and people working out. I felt such a buzz, and all those good feelings ran through me. I told Ali that I would step onto one of those treadmills one day.

On Sunday, I went to Ru's house to discuss fundraising. We began writing down ideas, names of people, names of companies, and by the end of the day we had a mini plan in place. We devised a campaign name #KeepingHope, together with a simple to-do list. During the next two days I nervously began with the list: I created a crowd-funding page, a Facebook page and I went to the bank to open a new account. I pulled together photos and wrote a campaign story board. All the practical things were in place. A few close friends and family members were ready for the campaign to go live. They were ready to begin sharing it with their respective networks.

Putting aside all the practical things I did during the day, I still grappled with the intangible. Am I worthy? Do

I deserve to live? Can I ask for help? Can I receive help? I talked through these themes with several mentors, and one night, as I went to bed, I quietly said yes to life. I chose to stay.

## REFLECTION

Hope is all I had left. I had family and friends who were ready to support a fundraising campaign, but I had to give it the go-ahead. I had several doubts, but I also believed in the possibilities. 'The little things' once more became important to me, following encounters with Roberta, Dave and Ali. Talking through and exploring my worthiness with long-term friends and mentors, Leonard and David, allowed me to get to a space where I felt worthy. The downward spiral reversed as I chose to keep hope; I chose to stay.

CHOICE FOURTEEN

# TO STAY

The morning finally came when I nervously activated my JustGiving page. My new Facebook page was rather lonely as I took a deep breath and shared my campaign with the world. My mind came up with endless possibilities for what could happen. At one extreme there was a fairy tale ending, with a wealthy individual saving the day and deciding to pay for the entire treatment. Another scenario was not raising anywhere near enough – a thought I didn't dwell on.

As soon as the campaign went live, I was blown away by the response.

My friend Maha was the first to donate and the first to share my page. She wrote: 'We've crossed many hurdles together since we've been best friends, Mo. This too shall pass!' Her words were comforting, and I knew I had several people on my team. Many others followed. People I knew, people I didn't know. They not only donated but shared the appeal, with heartfelt testimonials. Some donations were anonymous; some were left with messages of love, support and of prayers. I was humbled each time, as the notifications appeared on my phone multiple times a day. Each morning I would wake up to read message after message, and cry. There was so much love out there. All of a sudden I had #TeamMo, a community of people all over the world keeping an eye on the campaign and supporting me every step of the way.

There were supporters who organised local campaigns for me, campaigns at schools and universities, at community centres and at workplaces. There were cake sales, bouncy castles, movie nights and sponsored runs. I was overwhelmed by everything going on around me, for me.

My local mosque invited me to give a short talk to run a collection. I sat contemplating what I'd say while waiting for the imam to call me up. I thought about the times I had reached into my pockets to give to the mosque and all the times I had contributed to charitable causes. Now it was my turn to ask for help.

*'Salam (peace), my name is Momenul. I may look healthy but unfortunately I have late stage cancer. I had NHS treatment for a year, including chemo and a major operation, but that didn't work. My cancer is growing. We often hear of new breakthrough treatments in the news, and there is one that has a 70-80% chance of working for me called immunotherapy, but it's not on the NHS, and it costs too much. I've been told that it is Sunnah (a tradition of the Prophet) to seek treatment, that's why I am fundraising for £200,000, to give myself a chance. That's why I am here, to ask for your prayers, to ask*

*for your support. If you can donate whatever you can, I will be most grateful, thank you.'*

It only took a few moments to share, and following the prayer, buckets were sent around. Collections that day totalled more than £500. I was in awe.

Over the next few weeks and months I adapted this version of the talk, according to the time I was given at different mosques. I would take leaflets with me, detailing my crowdfunding link, allowing people to make donations electronically. Many people would come and speak to me after my talk, offering their support. Some would take my number and stay in touch. After one collection, a young man who looked like he was in his late teens/early twenties said: 'Bro, you're a soldier. Everyone should hear your story. I thought I had problems, but you have put things in perspective.' I continued to receive messages telling me I was 'inspiring', 'brave' and 'courageous'. I wasn't quite sure how to receive such kind words. It just felt like I was doing what I needed to do.

During the early part of my campaign I had ten days of radiotherapy spread across two weeks for the cancerous node in my neck. I had to juggle my activities between each shot. Some days I would go for the shot in the morning and then straight to an activity. On other days I would have the activity in the morning and a hospital visit later in the day. The nurses were full of support for my cause, as they clamped me down with an immobilisation mask to safely zap me with the powerful rays.

I would soon become a 'local celebrity', a term coined by my friends. I was stopped in the street by well-wishers. 'Are you Mo?', 'Are you the brother with cancer?', 'Are you the guy fundraising?' People were donating and were also following my progress.

My story was featured in the local newspapers and then in the mainstream media. I began speaking to journalists with more frequency. My MP Keir Starmer's communication with the Department of Health was picked up by the Evening Standard and then ITV London. I spent a morning filming at the hospital together with Ru and my oncologist, and the footage was broadcast on the 6pm news.

With no support coming from the government, Keir invited me to the Houses of Parliament for a reception event to raise further awareness. It felt surreal having my own event in the historic building, with my family, friends and supporters. I delivered an emotional speech, sharing how vulnerable the process had made me become, as well as my desire to help others.

I continued to get out of my comfort zone and in front of TV cameras when Sheikh Madani invited me on to his live TV show on a Bangladeshi channel to raise awareness. When I was in Makkah, he had said he would give me his full support and this was his way of doing that. We went on air at 10.30pm on a Sunday night for a 90-minute slot, but the phone lines were so busy the producers kept us on until 1am. We received call after call, with people expressing their sadness and pledging to donate.

The calls continued to come. I was invited to two other Bangladeshi TV channels on the Sky platform; Channel S and Bangla TV, for live appeals. My friends volunteered in the call centre, taking non-stop calls and hearing heartfelt stories of viewers, who were also affected by cancer and wanted to help save my life.

## REFLECTION

In all honesty, I have not fully absorbed this period of my life. It feels surreal to even be writing these words. I chose to be vulnerable and I chose to put my ego and pride to one side, and asked for help. The help was given to me in abundance, and I continue to receive the support with gratitude and love. As I chose to stay, I ultimately chose love.

# CHOICE FIFTEEN

# LOVE

Beginning the fundraising was daunting, but once it began I threw myself into it. There was no 'how to' book on fundraising. I just did whatever felt right and went wherever I was called to go. During the process I have been honoured to meet some incredible people and hear some humbling stories.

One morning, I read a Facebook message from a guy called Alex. It read something like this: 'Hi Mo, you don't know me. My name is Alex, I'm a friend of a friend of a friend… Stephanie [his girlfriend] and I heard your story and want to help. We have decided to do a cycle trek from the south of New Zealand to the north.' I couldn't believe a complete stranger would do something so extreme for me. They later explained to me that they had been travelling for over a year, and many people had helped them along the way, so they decided to pay it forward. I followed their updates across social media during the fifty days it took them to make that challenging journey, raising almost £5,000 towards the cause.

On another occasion, I went into my local pharmacy, which was running a collection for me. I regularly pop in to collect my prescription medicine and to share my updates with Nikita. That morning, she told me about a conversation she'd had with a homeless woman. The woman had come in for some painkillers and had stopped to read my story, which was displayed on the counter. She then reached into her pocket, grabbed some coins and put them on the counter. 'I want to be part of the campaign,' she said. Nikita said that she would put the coins in, on her behalf, but the woman said, 'No, it has to be my coins.' As I heard these words, I was humbled to the core. I was lost for words. Someone whom I would have judged to have nothing gave away her coins for me. Once more, I felt the love of strangers. I asked if Nikita knew her name but she didn't. I asked her to take down the woman's name and take a picture if she ever came in again.

One afternoon, after I collected my nephew from school and took him to the playground for a kick about, we were approached by a school kid on a bicycle. 'Are you the person who wasn't well?' he asked. 'I've been waiting to meet you, how are you?' He then asked if he could take a selfie, wished me well and moved on. These moments when people in my local community recognise me and ask how I am, are common. I always feel honoured and blessed that people not only supported me during my campaign, but continue to care about my wellbeing.

I have been blessed to hear many stories of people finding out about my campaign and deciding to help. The daughter of one man I met at a mosque heard my story and decided to run a collection of her own. She approached parents at her Saturday school and asked whether they would contribute. Through the process she raised over £200. Together with her dad, she came to drop off the money to me.

Some of the stories weren't about money, either. Thomas, the son of my friend Nicola, decided to request a prayer for me at school. He said, 'My friend Mo is unwell, can we say a prayer?' The class prayed for me. Afterwards, some children went up to him and said, 'We didn't know Mo Farah was ill, but we prayed for him. We hope he gets better.' These are stories that will stay with me forever.

Then there was another Alex from a production company who met up with me to discuss a possible documentary to raise awareness of health issues and the lack of access to certain medication on the NHS. Through the conversation, I told him about my love of Tottenham Hotspur and how going to games was difficult. The previous time I'd gone, my knees locked up and I struggled to walk. Without my knowing, Alex got in touch with the club, and a week later I was speaking with Tracey, who looks after Spurs Wishes. She offered me and four of my friends/ family a VIP experience at a live match. The kindness of strangers was, again, overwhelming.

There were some very challenging days along the way, too, when I questioned what I was doing. One of the most difficult days of my life – and I've had a few that I've shared in this book – was when my good friend Jack knocked on my door. It was around 10am, and I thought he had popped over for one of our regular catch-ups. Jack, struggling to get words out said, 'It's not a long visit, Mo.' He had some terrible news (I am actually feeling the chills as I write this here and the tears are coming as they did that morning). 'Barbara has died,' he said. Barbara was his wife, and I had seen her only the previous week, when she had proposed various ideas and had drafted letters to send to organisations, including Tottenham Hotspur (she also was a Spurs fan) to support our fundraising campaign.

Jack went on to say that they were asking people to donate to my campaign instead of giving flowers. Such a gesture of love made my heart well up even more. Even in death, Barbara gave to life. I didn't know what to say. I gave Jack a hug, just the way he had given me a hug when he found out about my cancer. Barbara, you are forever in our memories, and I wish you were still with us. As the fundraising began you said to me: 'If anyone can do this, you can.' Thank you, Barbara, I love you.

Barbara was right. Within the first month of my campaign, #TeamMo had raised a staggering £60,000, which allowed me to start the treatment. By the second month we'd raised £100,000, and by the time we had reached £185,000, we were no longer actively fundraising anymore. With the love of thousands of people from all over the world I was given a chance to save my life.

I went on to have sixteen cycles of immunotherapy, one every three weeks, spread out over a period of a year. I had CT scans every four cycles. After the first scan, I was told my tumours had reduced. When I looked at the results, the percentage difference was incredible. Some tumours had shrunk by 70%, others by 30%. I was relieved but cautious. After so much bad news over the last year and a half, this was very encouraging. It made all the fundraising worth it. Follow-up scans continued to show small reductions in size, until they were stable. My energy levels increased and I even made trips to the gym to step on to the treadmill with Ali. I was able to drive again, and was making the most of my time by looking for ways to help others with cancer.

After a year of treatment, from June 2016 to May 2017, my oncologist decided to pause the treatment in line with the research studies. I have regular scans every eight weeks to monitor the tumours, and ten months on (March 2018) the disease is stable. I am very grateful.

## REFLECTION

Going out to fundraise was the most daunting decision of my life, but choosing to do so gave others a chance to reach out and help, and choose love themselves. My story, my campaign, became their campaign. I am overwhelmed by the love, support and care I received, and I am grateful every single day that I am still alive. I wanted to 'live a life worth living' and now I want to help others too.

# SECTION TWO

# LESSONS

# LIFE – THERE IS MEANING IN EVERYTHING, EVEN IN SUFFERING

*'The meaning of life is to give life meaning.'*
**Viktor E. Frankl**

When I visited my friend and mentor Dr Kim with my cancer diagnosis, which I had received just a few hours earlier, I was devastated. At this stage we didn't know the exact plan of action because the experts were awaiting a multi-disciplinary team (MDT) meeting to discuss the way forward.

I was fearful, in shock and I didn't know what to do or what lay ahead of me. What I did have, however, were two questions I wanted help in answering:

What does this diagnosis mean?
Will I choose to stay?

A week after the MDT, the cancer specialist gave his expert opinion that I had a 'small chance of success.'

The prognosis was bleak and I was distraught. Dr Kim's words, 'You are more powerful than the words of any doctor,' gave me hope, and, in hindsight, this was exactly what I needed to hear.

Instead of the words 'I have a small chance of success' playing on loop in my head for the foreseeable future and being the repeat line in conversations, I was given the alternative option: 'I am more powerful than the words of any doctor.'

Words have meaning, and meaning has power to transform. If I had followed the 'small chance' thoughts it might have become a self-fulfilling prophecy – a phenomenon I learned about in sociology classes. Instead, following the 'I am more powerful' route gave me the will power to do my best each day. It gave me a sense of responsibility.

Dr Kim reminded me of my two questions, which then became my focus.

Cancer was about to change everything in my life and I wanted to find meaning. As a strong believer in everything happening for a reason, I wanted to find deeper meaning for my cancer and my life. Inspired by Viktor E. Frankl's Man's Search For Meaning, an account of how some prisoners survived concentration camps, it now became my very own search for meaning, a question of how I would survive a death sentence.

Regular conversations with Dr Kim enabled that exploration for meaning to begin. We met in person, we chatted online, we communicated through emails and messages. He was true to his words, when he said he 'would walk side by side, every step of the way' with me.

The search took me to 1985, when I was two and my dad died. He flew to Bangladesh in the hope for herbal remedies for his bowel cancer. The cancer that he had kept hidden from his family and friends was the same cancer I had. Only thirty years later, on the eve of 2015, I was doing things differently to my dad. I was sharing my cancer experience with the world. While he was alone, I had a loving support network around me.

Going through my ordeal, I felt closer to my dad than I had ever felt before. There was a lot of meaning for me; I always said I never got to know my dad, but I was going through a similar experience, with similar fears, yet taking a different approach. I now know my dad.

During my primary school years, the 'tummy ache' I often pretended to have, which meant my mum picked me up early, had now manifested in reality. It was only twenty-five years later that I was able to open up to my mum and tell her about the childhood emotional pain I felt. This in turn led to my mum telling me about the 'family curse' story that had passed on from generation to generation. The mother and children from the story in the 1800s are still alive in my thoughts, and their lives have meaning, even after all these years, as I honour them and pray for their souls.

As my cancer experience has unfolded, I've had the privilege of sharing my story across many platforms and through various media outlets. I continue to meet people who take inspiration from my words and story, many of whom are cancer patients themselves, and have embarked on their own daunting fundraising campaigns. Cancer threatened to take my life away, yet it has given me the gift of appreciating every single day and has allowed me to be of service to others.

I now fully appreciate that there is a definite meaning in my cancer and my suffering. I continue to find new levels of depth and connection, and I am mindful that I may never know about the ripple effects that my story has. If I am ever lucky enough to hear about one of those ripples, I would be extremely humbled.

I do know that nothing is ever wasted and that there is meaning in everything, even in death.

## EXERCISE: HOW TO FIND MEANING IN CHALLENGING TIMES

1. Would you like to explore meaning in your life?

The first step is to set an intention. I would encourage you to acknowledge that there is meaning and that you will go deep to find it. If you are going through a challenge or suffering from pain from the past, you might want to find meaning in these. Sometimes you can do this by asking the question, 'What does this mean?' and then waiting patiently for answers to be revealed.

2. After setting an intention, there is an active process.

Ask the question every single day and affirm: 'I am willing to find meaning in this.' If answers aren't obvious, continue to ask every day. Look for clues, listen to your instinct and pay attention to the words other people say.

3.   Keep a journal of any insights you get.

Go back to those moments and see the trajectory of the incidents. What choices did you make as a result? Who did you meet? What changes did you make? It can be an emotional process, but trust me, when you find your meaning there will be a huge shift.

4.   Talk to wise and trusted people about your experiences.

Sometimes this can provoke questions that you've never asked or thought about, and can lead to the switch that turns the lightbulb on. I've heard the phrase 'God speaks through others'. If you're not comfortable with the word God, replace it with another word, but listen and look for answers in the most unexpected places.

I have a story related to clues.

My friend Dasha asked me to read a book called The Fault In Our Stars, by John Green, six months before my diagnosis. I had never heard of it and politely said I would. So many books have been recommended to me over the years and it was unlikely that I would go out to buy this as I wasn't in the mood to read any books. I was finding life a challenge at this point. But it was also the summer holidays for my nephews. I went into a book shop to buy some activity books for them to keep them occupied. As I was looking at the children's books on the shelves, I heard something fall behind me. I turned around to see a toy had fallen over, but I also noticed The Fault In Our Stars had been misplaced on the children's display table. I smiled, took a picture and then bought it.

I began reading the book during Ramadan to find it was about two cancer patients. The first line read: 'That's the thing about pain. It demands to be felt.' It was during the end of Ramadan that I became sick and started developing symptoms. The pain at the time stopped me from completing the book.

It could be said that I didn't follow up at the time on the deeper significance of this encounter and associate my pain with cancer, but looking back, the clues were always there. I just didn't notice.

## LESSON TWO

# LIFE'S PAIN HAS SOMETHING TO TELL US

*'That's the thing about pain. It demands to be felt.'*
**John Green, The Fault In Our Stars**

That morning in October 2014, the words 'We feel pain, we take pain killers, and the pain goes away' were etched in my mind. The nurse couldn't have been more wrong. Each set of tablets increased in potency over the following six weeks until I was finally diagnosed. The pain was excruciating and affected my sleep, my work, and my life overall.

Now, yes, it is possible for tablets to reduce the pain and perhaps even get rid of the pain just as the nurse suggested. I am not proposing I should never take them. My understanding, though, is that the tablets are designed to numb the pain, while the root cause(s) remain, unless, of course, those causes are explored and treated. Sometimes, the cause of the pain is obvious, such as from an injury or a lack sleep, but it is not always so clear.

Sometimes, the causes can be traced back to lifestyle, diet or to an injury, but sometimes deep introspection is needed. Take the example of a lack of sleep causing headaches. Maybe tablets can ease the pain and allow you to function with the day ahead. Over time, however, that headache may grow in intensity and the pain killers will need to get stronger and stronger. The body is requesting sleep and rest, but by taking pain killers we decide not to listen continuing to perform at the same intensity and over time, this can result in a more serious illness.

While I was having an infusion of immunotherapy, my uncle came to visit me and told me some terrible news about one of his friends who had been operated on the previous day. His friend had been going to the doctors for over a year complaining of headaches, but was always sent away with tablets. The medics said he had a migraine and didn't carry out further investigations. It was when he collapsed at home and was taken to A&E that they found a huge tumour in the brain and performed surgery that lasted ten hours. His friend sadly died a few months later.

## MY CANCER SIGNS

If I go back a few months to July 2014, it was the holy month of Ramadan when I was fasting from approximately

3.30am to 9pm, almost 17 hours a day. Towards the end of Ramadan, with a few more days to go, I vomited at work. I had been fasting for more than twenty years and I do not remember ever vomiting. I visited the doctor and between us we put it down to the fasting. My sleep patterns were disrupted, I was dehydrated and had low energy levels because I didn't eat during the fasting hours. With hindsight, this was a sign something wasn't quite right.

Other signs included random abdominal pain while I was at work. I would be in meetings when all of a sudden I would feel a sharp stab in my belly. I would get up, go to the toilet or walk about. I know colleagues were concerned but I didn't think it was serious. The pain would always go away.

In addition to the stomach cramps, I would have loose stools, again feedback from my body, but I didn't think it was serious.

Physically, I carried on with my running and training routine, which was my way of numbing the pain. I thought that because I could run 5km in less than 20 minutes, and 10km in 40 minutes, I was healthy. I also didn't smoke or drink. When my running times were five minutes slower than my personal best, and my running partner, JD, lapped me on the track, I put it down to poor form on my part and to JD increasing his fitness.

What I have learned is that pain is trying to tell us something. It is a call for attention, and in the case of cancer-induced pain, it is a wakeup call, the body's last resort for help.

It was only in October 2014, when the pain reached unbearable levels, that I made frequent visits to the doctors. I then noticed I had lost weight significantly when the doctor asked me to step on to the scales. I had dropped 5kgs in what must have been a few months without any dieting. All this, together with being told that I was unusually anaemic, signalled that something might be wrong. The fact that I needed to put on a belt for jeans that I previously didn't need to, was completely missed.

I missed all the warning signs that led to my advanced cancer diagnosis. Although, once diagnosed, I still had opportunities to listen to the pain.

In the darkest hour one night, I woke up with abdominal pain that I have no words to describe. Excruciating, unbearable and unimaginable have already been used. This night, the pain was too much. I paced around my room in the dark, I sat on the toilet seat, but the pain wouldn't budge. In desperation I fell to my knees bedside, with my face in the duvet. I began pleading with the pain. What do you want? What do you want me to do? And then, almost instantly, miraculously, I felt enveloped by love. I felt comfort as the pain eased in that moment. It was like the pain was waiting for me to connect with it.

The cancer became an invitation to begin an exploration for meaning. I became aware that the emotional pain I'd felt from the past was being bottled up in my gut. Instead of communicating about the things that had upset me over the last three decades, I was storing them up. The physical pain was now allowing me to release old wounds, and, in the process, encourage me to express new upsets as and when they occurred. Many of these I have shared in previous chapters.

## EXERCISE: HOW TO LISTEN TO YOUR PAIN

Disclaimer: If you are in pain, please seek medical help.

The first step is to acknowledge that there is pain and that there are root causes.

With so many stimulants in the world it is difficult to tune into our bodies. It is important to find time to be still, be quiet, and be with the pain.

I would encourage you to talk to the pain and to ask it questions. Put your hand on the pain, and be present. Focus as much attention as you can on the pain and feel it.

Listen for answers. The answers may come in subtle ways.

I would also encourage you to think about when the pain began to surface.

- Can you remember the initial signs? Think back to when the pain began.

- When did it begin? Is there a date you can associate it with? A month or a year, perhaps?

- What was going on in your life at the time? What was going on in the following areas of your life: work, relationship, family, finances, social, health and spiritual?

- What was your life like at the time? Who were the people you were spending your time with? What were the projects you were working on?

- How did you spend your time?

Some of these questions will trigger your memory and help you get some answers.

Working with a practitioner can be extremely powerful.

I developed shoulder and knee pain so I went to see Chris, who is a movement therapist, to see if he could help me. A few simple questions later, I traced the pain back to when the medical team inserted a port above my chest, which was stitched underneath my skin. The port allowed drug infusions to be applied quickly without the need to connect a cannula to me every time. At the time of incision, the nurse said the ports can sometimes get twisted, which would require a trip to the hospital. With that warning I began suppressing my natural arm movements to protect the port. When

I went to sleep, I'd position my body to protect the right shoulder.

When Chris assessed me, he observed that I was not using the lower spine to its maximum range. This meant the pelvis wasn't being used as it was designed, impacting my knees, which also had an impact on my shoulder. I was given an exercise routine to regain range of the lower spine, and within weeks my knees and shoulders were pain free.

Once more, I stress, if you are in pain, please seek medical help.

LESSON THREE

# HAVING A VISION –
# A LIFE OF NO REGRETS

*'Those who have a "why" to live, can bear with
almost any "how".'*
**Viktor E. Frankl**

In my ten years of going to personal development seminars, I've heard several speakers say something along the lines: 'If the why is big enough, the how will find its way,' or 'Be clear on the why and the how will sort itself out.' The challenge is always discovering the 'why'.

It was in July 2014, five months before the cancer diagnosis, when I went to visit Dr Kim. At the time, I was frustrated with life. Patterns were repeating themselves at work; it was the third restructure I was involved in within a ten-year period and there was gossiping, uncertainty and many political battles, which left me drained. On a personal level, I was questioning my identity, something that was triggered by my equality and diversity work. There were moments when I inexplicably broke down, just thinking about 'who I was'. I had severed a number of friendships in a short period of time, cutting people out because of my 'all or nothing' mindset. I allowed friendships to end without communicating what was really bothering me. There were just too many things to process on top of the physical symptoms, which I hadn't taken seriously.

Upon hearing my list of troubles, Dr Kim brought out some blank sheets of paper, together with colouring pens. It was most unexpected. He induced me into a state of presence and focus, and then said: 'If today was the last day of your life, what would you have achieved and experienced to make it a fulfilled life?' He asked me to draw my life of no regrets. That was my task as I picked up the pens and began drawing. When I stopped, the page was made up of images, symbols and words for what my life of no regrets would look like. 'Leave a legacy' was written across the top in bold. It was clear I wanted to leave a mark, to 'make a dent', as Steve Jobs once said. I just had no idea 'how' I would go about my global vision, but at this stage it didn't matter. 'The "how" will find itself,' Dr Kim reminded me. As the session came to an end, he asked me to do further work on each item on my page.

I did begin to do the work in the following months as he suggested, but with the new term beginning at university, my job took all my attention. During this time, my health struggles began.

The next time I went to see Dr Kim was in December, after my diagnosis, and I had forgotten about 'my picture'. It was the last thing on my mind. Yet my picture was very much at the forefront of Dr Kim's mind. Every time I saw him, he would bring a copy out of my file and remind me to look at my picture, to feel it, to live it, to see myself living my life of no regrets. I wasn't sure why he kept telling me to do this, but I didn't question him. For me, the vision looked remote as I surrendered purely to staying alive.

It was a year later that I asked him about his fascination with 'the picture'. He reminded me of the instructions he had given. 'If today was the last day of your life...' The profound significance of my picture then hit me. Every time I looked at it, felt it, was it, I was subconsciously holding my vision. I was seeing a future with me in it. It was an anchor to live for; it was my reason for being, for carrying on, for choosing to stay. Only I wasn't conscious of this at the time.

It then occurred to me that I was living 'my life of no regrets', as I continued to take each day as it came. I was slowly working through each part of the puzzle.

I am speaking my truth, I am writing my book, I am creating the curriculum for the 'School of Hope'. I don't know what 'legacy' I will leave behind, or whether I will make that 'dent'. I just know that my story has reached several people in many parts of the world, and if I work on each piece of the picture, I will have lived a life no regrets.

# EXERCISE: HOW TO FIND YOUR VISION

I would suggest going back to being a child.

- What were the things you wanted to be?

- Are there themes that connect?

- What were you passionate about? What are you passionate about now?

I remember I wanted to be a news reporter as a child. I used to role play and pretend to read the news. Now, later in life, my aim is to speak my truth, to share my story across various platforms.

- If money were no object and you could achieve anything you wanted to do, what would you do?

  Undistracted, be clear about your vision. Quiet the mind, close your eyes, take deep breaths, meditate and play some inspiring music. Allow yourself to write, draw and visualise. Whatever you feel inspired by, get it down. Then look at your picture, read your statement, and visualise yourself living that vision.

This is the first part of finding your vision. You might want to go back and refine this process as the days, months and years go by. You might want to add to your vision or take things out that no longer inspire.

Crucially, the second part is to act. Remember the 'how' will look after itself, but it still requires action.

There is no linear path. There will be ups and downs and obstacles along the way. I would suggest reframing the obstacles or challenges that you face. I see them as a test to see how serious I am about achieving a goal. For example, shall I make that call? Send that email? Attend an event?

You never know who you will meet along the path. Learn to communicate the different parts of your vision and be brave in asking for help. One of my mentors, Daniel Priestley, says: 'You get what you pitch for, and you're always pitching.'

- How are you showing up? What are you pitching?

  Holding the vision closely in your mind's eye will help you remember your reasons for being. If there's one thing you are inspired to do that one day, just do that one thing. That will be liberating your future.

I often sit quiet and still in the morning, take a few deep breaths and say the following:

- Where would you have me go?

- What would you have me do?

- What would you have me say?

- And to whom?

I then patiently listen for answers in the form of intuition, meeting requests, and I follow up on ideas and instincts as they appear. Amazing things can happen, but it requires action.

My fundraising campaign was public; I asked for help, and I was asked to attend several meetings, events and do things for the first time, including media appearances.

There were days when I was in pain or I was tired and wanted an extra hour in bed, but I would remember my vision and ask myself the question, 'Will doing this activity bring me closer to my vision?' If the honest answer was 'yes, it will', I would act accordingly. It was during these days that I went on to share my vision and attract new people to my life to support me.

LESSON FOUR

# HONOUR
# THE PAST

*'The unexamined life is not worth living.'*
**Socrates**

In the previous lesson I spoke about the importance of having a vision for the future, one that truly inspires you to live a life of no regrets. This is something that helped me get through each day.

In this lesson I talk about the importance of releasing the energy from past events, built up in the form of emotions, which may include upsets, regrets, shame and guilt. Equally, there will be positive emotions from good times, and it's about honouring and celebrating those too.

When I got the diagnosis and the prognosis it shook me to the core. I wasn't sure how long I had to live. I didn't want to die with potential upsets from the past remaining in the ether.

There were situations and people with whom I had unresolved issues. I wanted to release the hurt and make amends. I also wanted to heal all the wounds that were still held inside me, so that I could clear away the past but also honour it. I wanted to forgive myself and anyone else I was feeling resistance against, and in the process take away any potential learning.

I made a list of people with whom I felt I had hurt and let down. I got in touch with them and apologised sincerely for my actions and asked for their forgiveness and their prayers. Making the phone calls, sending the emails and messages felt liberating. A weight of burden and pain had been lifted.

I then made a list of significant events from the past that still held an emotional charge.

With each event, I decided to give empathy to myself.

I picked up the two-year-old baby that was me, and held him in my arms. I remembered the pain he felt when his dad never returned, which he kept hidden from the world. I told my two-year-old self that everything was okay, that he was loved, and that he would understand the meaning of this pain when he was ready.

Likewise, I spoke to my dad, forgave him for leaving and felt empathy for the pain he must have been in. I felt closer to him than ever before. I let go of the abandonment I had felt for a large part of my life, and appreciated how difficult life must have been for him. With everything I have experienced with cancer, his choices now had context. It is likely the doctors in the UK gave up on him, advanced treatments being a distant dream. In keeping hope, perhaps he went in search of alternative herbal remedies.

I shared the truth with my mum about my pretend tummy aches, about all the stories I made up because I was afraid of losing her too and being an orphan. Once more, I felt liberated to release the guilt inside me that I had harboured for almost twenty five years.

I went back to the village story; 'the curse', where the mother was separated from her two sons. The story that has been passed down through the generations and now to me. I prayed for their souls. I prayed for the forgiveness of the men involved in their stories, and by sharing their story publicly I hope to pay tribute to them in honouring them, in giving meaning to their lives all these years later.

As I went down my list, I forgave myself for all the times I didn't speak my truth, or take action. The times I let myself or others down.

I thanked myself for all the times I came out of my comfort zone and made myself vulnerable, like when I stood for election. I almost fainted during one talk, but I carried on to eventually get elected. That difficult year ended up being character building, and led to a whole new career.

I thanked myself for the compassion I had, for the desire to help others, whether that was to help students through my eventual profession, or to help the less fortunate through my contributions over the years.

There was a time when I found myself in a spiral of debt. The financial situation was so desperate, I was counting the pennies in a money jar before going shopping. I thanked myself for bravely asking for guidance, even though I felt shame and embarrassment about the situation. Ultimately, this ask was the trigger for a plan of action. I became disciplined in my spending and saving habits. In a short few years I was able to turn the situation around and be in a position to offer guidance to others in similar difficulties.

I also made peace with myself for missing all the signs of cancer. I know that the path I've been on has been full of pain and suffering, yet equally there has been a lot of joy and meaning. All I can do now is to be present with my whole body and pay attention to any pain that arises and take appropriate action.

I made peace with who I was, and who I am.

I affirmed that:

- I am enough
- I do enough
- I have enough
- My presence is enough

## EXERCISE: SUGGESTIONS FOR HONOURING THE PAST

Make a list of all the significant moments in your life, both positive and negative – moments that hold an emotional charge.

- With the positive moments, what made them feel good? What did you do to make them happen? Give yourself the appreciation for serving yourself.

- With the negative moments, do they still bring an emotional charge? If so, what is the charge for each one?

- Does holding onto this serve you? Will letting this go serve you better?

To release emotional charge, I advise writing about it, and speaking to a trained professional. Here's a spiritual practice I often do:

1. Get in tune with the emotion. What is the feeling? The temptation might be to ignore or push the feeling away. But stay with it, and ask it what it wants you to hear.

2. Be objective. It's easy to become judgemental and be upset by having negative feelings, but these feelings are valid. Give yourself compassion. Remind yourself 'I am enough, I do enough, I have enough, my presence is enough.'

3. Find the corresponding need for the emotion.

4. Once you know the need, take the appropriate action. This might involve having a conversation

with someone (I talk more about this in the next chapter).

5. Meditate: focus on the issue and go into a meditation with the intention to release the charge. I often say, 'God, I hand this issue over to you.'

It is my belief that everything from the past has the ability to teach us something, if we look for the lessons.

Now this practice didn't work for me straight away or in one sitting; it developed over several weeks and months. In fact, my work continues, as there will always be fresh upsets. What I've learned is that it's best to deal with the upsets as soon as they occur.

I am still learning to find healthy ways, and am acknowledging that I have a way to go. There was a recent unhealthy occasion in the bank. I was in the midst of a flurry of fundraising activity, and I had an appointment booked with a doctor while waiting at the bank. The cashier asked me to take a seat and that they would be a minute with my documents. A minute turned to fifteen minutes, and then twenty minutes. During this time, I was feeling irate inside, and this feeling continued to build up. I had an appointment to get to and I had no time to waste. I didn't know how to express my frustration, and just began loudly shouting: 'Why am I waiting?' This was out of character. Immediately, someone came out of an office. It happened to be the area manager, who calmed me down and allowed me to explain and release the frustration. I would never have imagined causing such a scene, and I later described it as a 'diva fit'.

# LIVING IN THE NOW

*'The past is history, the future is a mystery,*
*and the present is a gift'*
**Kung Fu Panda**

It is easy to hold onto regrets, guilt and/or shame from the past. That's why in the previous lesson, I talked about honouring the past and letting go of emotions from situations that don't serve our healing. Living with a life threatening illness means the future is always uncertain. I've created many stories in my head about what might happen based on fears, some imagined, some rational.

In this lesson, I share the importance of living in the moment as often as possible, which includes being true to our fears, as well as our wishes, hopes and dreams, as they come up.

Many people tell me that I am a positive person, inspiring even, and these words mean a lot. Yet, I don't want people to have a false impression of me. I have my fair share of feeling down, and at times I feel like I can no longer be bothered to carry on with the so-called 'fight'. During these times, the last thought on my mind is to take a picture, or share the agony with a post across my social media channels. No one sees the times I wake up at night in tears or with pain. The truth is, I have lots of negative thoughts but I don't dwell on them.

What I've learned to do is be present. In these moments, I slow down and try to acknowledge what I'm feeling. I get in touch with my emotions. I question what I am feeling. Am I feeling angry? Am I sad? Am I upset? Am I scared? Am I anxious? The range of possible feelings are vast, yet the closer I am to the exact feeling, the closer I am to knowing the corresponding need I have. Once I am aware of the need, I can then begin to do something about it. It then becomes a process of finding the next action or request.

One of the scariest moments I had was when I got a call from the hospital telling me that they had detected a blood clot in my lungs, a 'pulmonary embolism', after a CT scan. At that precise moment I felt resigned. I remember the sigh it brought, along with the tears. I was fearful because I thought blood clots were serious (and they are). I sent a few messages to close friends sharing my concerns. I was already feeling the effects of chemotherapy, and this was unexpected and brought a lot more uncertainty, but I was true to my feelings rather than denying them. The fear in this case was rational;

the doctors had asked me to go to the hospital straight away because of the seriousness of the situation. All I could do was go to the hospital and wait for the doctors to assess me. I was lucky the blood clot had been detected and I could be admitted immediately. I remained in hospital for over a week and I was given blood thinning injections, which I took every day for eighteen months. Thankfully, the blood clot is no longer there.

Anyone who has spent time with me over the past couple of years may have noticed that I put my hand on my belly occasionally. Sometimes people ask if I'm okay, with a look of concern. I am doing it to check my stoma, making sure that there are no leaks and seeing if the bag needs emptying. One evening, I was out with friends when I decided to check my stoma. I immediately knew something wasn't right. I could feel a prolapse through my stoma. Parts of my bowel were coming through, a bit like a hernia. It wasn't painful but it needed my attention. I went home immediately, removed my stoma bag and lay back on my bed to try to relax as previously advised.

The first time it happened I was at home and was scared, as I had no idea what was happening. I called the emergency oncology number, took a picture of it and sent an email to my nurse and doctor. The prolapse went back in quite quickly and I was told to go straight to A&E if the colour turned purple, which would signify a loss of blood supply and would need surgery. This time round, it was taking longer to go back down. I made the same phone call to the emergency number to let them know, and then called my friend, asking him to be on standby in case I needed to go to A&E.

In each of these health scares, I was able to tune into the moment and focus. Nothing else came close to being on my mind. I was truly present, which allowed me to navigate the moment by staying calm while acknowledging the seriousness of the situation. I was then able to take the next step.

It is easy to worry in moments like this, particularly as the mind is trying to fill in the blanks. Many people I've met who have cancer have bouts of 'scanxiety', when waiting for scan results creates a sense of anxiety. I'm no different. I have become accustomed to getting my results from my oncologist within a few days. After one particular scan, however, there was no phone call or a reply to my message. After a week had gone by and I still had no news, I began fearing the worst. 'He's not calling me because it's bad news,' was one train of thought. Yet, what really happened was that my oncologist was out of the country and couldn't access the computer system and both my cancer specialist nurses were away. They would have ordinarily sent him the results. During that time I was creating a script in my head that fuelled unnecessary negativity.

## EXERCISE: HOW TO LIVE IN THE MOMENT

To help cultivate a state of presence I have developed a set of daily rituals. This includes mindfulness exercises, such as meditation, conscious breathing and gratitude lists.

I also carry out purposeful movement exercises where each motion is carried out with focus and attention on the body, the breath and my thoughts in the moment. Qi Gong is something I have found helpful.

Whenever I feel an emotional charge, I get clear on the emotion. Every emotion corresponds to a need. When the emotion is positive, needs are being fulfilled. Contrarily, if it's a negative emotion, needs are not being met.

If it's fear I have, I check to see if it's based on reality or if it's an imagined script I've created in my head. If it is a real fear, I then talk to the appropriate people and act accordingly. Not talking or acting on the fear results in a space of future worry and anxiety, which inevitably takes you away from the moment.

Being true to myself very much allows me to stay in the moment as often as possible. Being in denial takes me away from the moment.

Being still and quiet and focusing on your breath while noticing small movements is the quickest way to become present.

- Keep a diary for a few days and monitor your levels of presence

- Make a list of distractions that take you off track from whatever you are working on

- Do certain thoughts about the future or the past take up your energy?

Becoming aware of these distractions and thoughts is powerful in building strategies to stay present.

I discovered what it meant to be focused through my work with Anastasia, a behavioural analyst. I was on a programme to better apply my mind using the latest research in neuroscience. One of the exercises was to play a brain training game, which tested my memory, focus and speed. My goal was to get 100% accuracy each time and improve my best score. What I discovered was that the smallest distraction, such as a text message notification, someone calling my name, or music from a TV advert, was enough to put me off track and not get the desired result. I realised how easy it is to lose the moment, but this also showed me how focused I can be, if I am mindful about distractions.

# SELF-CARE COMES FIRST

*'How you treat yourself is how you are inviting the world to treat you.'*
**Unknown**

*'Self-care is not selfish. You can't serve from an empty vessel.'*
**Eleanor Brown**

Self-care became a buzz word for me as my desire for health and healing continued to flow. The more I kept talking about the topic with anyone who listened, the more I noticed articles and blogs about self-care. I came to realise that there are various levels of self-care, and I've grouped them into four levels or layers. Each layer builds on the previous, and if the first isn't in place it is very unlikely that the more advanced levels will be achieved.

The first level is around personal hygiene. It is what we learn as children and will no doubt be automatic for the majority of people. I'm talking about tasks such as regular bathing or showering, wearing clean clothes, changing underwear and socks and brushing teeth both morning and night. Activities which would ordinarily need no thought or prompting, which become part of everyday routines.

After my diagnosis, I went from a regimen of waking up early to get ready for an hour-and-a-half commute to work, to having no external pressure to get out of bed on a daily basis, unless I had a morning appointment at the hospital. There were moments during my cancer when I did not carry out even the basics of personal hygiene. Drugged up with chemo for days, the last thing I wanted to do was have a shower. I just didn't have the energy. Shaving became a chore with a PICC line connected to my arm, and I had no real reason to look professional. During some very dark days I felt like a caveman. I felt dirty on the inside; I was dirty on the outside.

Life got so dark that the basics of self-care were neglected. I know I'm not the only one to have experienced this, and it got worse. When I learned that the NHS would not fund my treatment, I went into a state of depression. I stayed in my pyjamas for a number of days, which felt like weeks. Time stood still. I couldn't be bothered to brush my teeth at night. I was sitting in self-pity, unsure how long I had left to live. Relatives would come to see me, while I was rooted to the sofa watching a TV screen, not paying attention to what was on. It was only when the day came for a pre-planned catch up with Roberta, who was over from Brazil, that I decided to pull myself together and make an effort to go out, changing my pattern as I set out to fundraise.

Level 2 of self-care is about wellness habits that enrich us. Healthy food, water, exercise and having enough sleep are pillars of self-care, which provide vitality for everyday living. Eating foods that nourish, drinking fluid such as water and green juices that fuel, moving our bodies to energise and keep the blood circulating, and having enough sleep to renew are crucial for vitality and functionality.

It's easy to indulge and lose this balance. Sleep can be compromised by working late hours or watching a show or browsing a screen/device until it is almost time to wake up. A lack of sleep over a period of time can mean our bodies are not repairing and replenishing. It stops the parasympathetic nervous system from doing its job.

When it comes to food, it's not the one-off pizza or burger that contributes to bad health, but fast food when it becomes the everyday norm. Guidance is readily available but the rapid increase in obesity is concerning.

Our bodies and brains are made up of between 70-80% water, so drinking enough water is important for our blood to flow efficiently. Moving our bodies (safely) is equally important.

Level 3 of self-care is what I call the 'paradox of disconnecting and connecting' and involves disconnecting from the constant demands that are put upon us, including stimulation through social media, emails and messages. These distractions are constant, with notifications and 'ping' sounds grabbing our attention at unprecedented levels. Instead, we need to regularly and consciously make time for ourselves to quiet our minds, allowing for connection with ourselves on a spiritual level. This practice needs to be scheduled in and can take many forms: a walk through nature, meditation, prayer or even mindfulness exercises. It's about doing less, and allowing ourselves to just be.

As my awareness grew, I spent time in flotation tanks every two weeks. These are sensory-deprived tanks full of Epsom salt, which allowed my senses to rest. I also attended monthly rebirthing sessions, also known as breathwork, a healing type of breathing practice that enabled me to feel more connected to my body and more at peace. I began attending weekly Qi Gong classes, which allowed me to carry out very slow motions in sync with my breathing to keep me mindful and in the moment. I also had regular acupuncture sessions. There are many ways to do this level of self-care, but I repeat, this needs to be scheduled in.

What I found was that during these connected moments, my awareness and consciousness increased. At times, questions came to my mind that arose from unresolved issues from the past, or certain patterns of behaviour or patterns within relationships that I attracted or destroyed were flagged up. This is where the fourth layer of self-care comes in.

Level 4 is about having mentors to regularly talk to. It is not unusual to have a mentor in a professional working setting, but having a mentor for life may not be that common. According to a Sage study, in the UK 22% of small businesses make use of business mentors. I suspect the figure for individual mentors is significantly lower. Yet working with a mentor can help establish healthy boundaries in all aspects of our lives including relationships, and help us to learn from and release old issues. Having a level of support allows us to take on new behaviours or habits, which can be difficult.

I believe that once the four levels become habitual, we are then able to help others find their way in self-care, possibly by becoming a mentor.

Having this awareness of the different levels has been useful for me as I fluctuate between them. Living with cancer has never been a linear process, as there are bad days along the way. It's during those difficult times that I push myself to do the level one self-care practices, which in itself feels like an accomplishment. 'Take each day as it comes' is the mantra that comes to mind when I have a framework to benchmark myself against.

## EXERCISE: SELF-CARE AUDIT

### LEVEL 1: PERSONAL CARE

This is not intended to be patronising in any way. These are real struggles I went through during some of my darkest days when carrying these out felt like an achievement. Some of these I aimed to do daily, some weekly, and others, such as getting my hair trimmed, monthly.

Tasks such as:

- Personal hygiene, eg bathing or showering

- Oral hygiene: brushing morning and night, flossing

- Fingernail and hand care

- Toenail and foot care

- Shaving/grooming

- Hair care: cutting, brushing, washing

- Clothing: changing underwear and socks, laundry, changing the bedding

Depending on how physically able you are, you might need to ask for help. Local authorities and social services may be able to arrange a simple care package to help with some tasks. Likewise, charities may be able to help.

It is difficult to ask for help in these areas, but having open conversations with loved ones can help you to devise a plan.

Are there any other tasks I have missed?
What are some of the basic everyday tasks that you have challenges with?

SELF-CARE COMES FIRST

| Task | Daily | Weekly | Monthly |
|---|---|---|---|
| Bathing/ Showering | | | |
| Brushing | | | |
| Fingernails | | | |
| Toenails | | | |
| Hand care | | | |
| Foot care | | | |
| Brushing hair | | | |
| Washing hair | | | |
| Cutting hair | | | |
| Shaving | | | |
| Changing clothes | | | |
| Underwear | | | |
| Socks | | | |
| Laundry | | | |
| Bedding | | | |

## LEVEL 2: VITALITY

### Sleep

- How much sleep are you getting?

- Do you have a sleep routine?

- What can you do to prepare for a better night's sleep?

- Do you wake up feeling energised?

### Food

- What are your eating habits like?

- The government guidance is to eat more than five portions of fruit and vegetables a day. Are you doing this?

- How can you improve your food intake?

- What are your cravings?

### Exercise

- Are you getting exercise?

- Depending on your level of health, what practices are you doing? What practices can you begin to incorporate in your life?

- If you are at a point where you are not doing any exercise, can you start by walking, even if it's for a few minutes every day?

Always check with your doctor before starting any exercise, but tasks such as walking, gentle yoga, Tai Chi, Qi Gong are very simple to begin with.

Monitor your progress, and add to your routine as you develop. Dancing, jogging, or bouncing on a mini trampoline for even a few minutes a day improves levels of fitness. You can join a class or start from your bedroom.

**Water**

- How much water are you drinking each day?

- What can you do to increase hydration?

## LEVEL 3: CONNECTION

How much time and energy do you give for a deeper connection with yourself?

- What activities do you participate in that keep you relaxed and rejuvenated?

- Do you do these activities daily, weekly, monthly?

- What do you do for fun?

- What can you do daily, weekly or monthly?

- Are any of the activities in the table part of your schedule?

- What can you add to your schedule to give yourself this gift?

| Activity | Daily | Weekly | Monthly |
|---|---|---|---|
| Meditation | | | |
| Yoga | | | |
| Walk in nature | | | |
| Massage | | | |
| Journaling | | | |
| Disconnect from technology for set periods of time | | | |

| | | | |
|---|---|---|---|
| Conscious breathing | | | |
| Flotation tanks | | | |
| Rebirthing | | | |
| Qi Gong | | | |
| Tai Chi | | | |
| Dancing | | | |
| Acupuncture | | | |
| Prayer | | | |

## LEVEL 4: MENTORS

- Who is your mentor?

- Do you have more than one mentor?

- Whose advice and support would you find valuable?

- What sort of help would you look to your mentor(s) to provide?

# LIFE IS MOVEMENT

*'Movement is the song of the body.'*
**Vanda Scaravelli**

The surgery to remove my colon and cancer left me bed-ridden. I couldn't move for several days. The anaesthetic left my legs and upper body numb. The wound from the operation stretched from the top of the abdomen to the bottom, and was stapled together. The area was raw, weak and sensitive. My movement was extremely limited; I was unable to even pull myself up in the bed, I had a catheter collecting my urine and I had a stoma to collect my stools. The nurses would change my stoma, empty the catheter and would pull me up on the bed whenever I slid down from the pillow.

After more than a week of lying in the hospital bed, relying on others for help, it was time to regain some movement. The physiotherapists began to work with me to firstly sit up, then stand, and then to take a step. These initial movements were extremely tough, and I needed the support of the team for every motion. Soon it was time for me to take those first steps on my own, like a baby. The catheter was removed and I slowly regained some independence again.

My fascination for movement was alive. When I lacked mobility, my desire to move intensified. Taking a baby step approach, I appreciated the fact that I could sit up, stand and walk on my own. I was grateful that I could also stretch various parts of my body. I felt liberated in movement.

I became conscious of the power of simple movements, of how, from a standing position, lifting only my right big toe could move my left shoulder. Every part is connected to the whole.

After I began immunotherapy, I had a burst in energy, which took my exploration to deeper levels. I was able to go back to the gym for gentle sessions, which felt incredible. I was doing yoga exercises every day, I started Qi Gong lessons once a week and bounced on a rebounder (mini trampoline) at home. I felt alive.

Yet after a year of immunotherapy, the treatment was paused and my movements hit rock bottom once more. One of the side effects I began to experience was arthritis. It began with pain in one knee, then the other. Both feet followed with swelling, my hands became stiff and then my elbows became inflamed to the point where I was unable to walk or use my arms freely. I would be outside when all of a sudden my knees would lock, my feet would swell, and I'd struggle to get home.

When I attempted to lie down on the floor for an exercise, it would be extremely challenging as my hands were unable to hold any weight. When I was lying down on the floor, I couldn't turn to the side, left or right, and it was with great difficulty that I would get up. I would rely on using my elbow to leverage my body weight and then grab hold of a piece of furniture to get back up.

My movement routine was derailed, another low for me. My new question was: 'Why do we do anything?'

I felt like a baby with my inability to freely move around or even get up. I then began observing the development of a new born baby. I know the following description is simplistic, but it illustrates the point.

Babies start off in a lying position. They like to put their fingers in their mouths, and when they discover their feet, these too go into their mouths. That's the beginning of the exploration.

Then they begin rocking to either side and eventually turn on their bellies. They then get stuck in that position and soon learn to roll back. When they are on their bellies they see the world from a different angle. They begin to reach out to grab toys (or anything else) and in doing so, swim on the floor. They eventually begin to crawl.

They learn to sit up, to crawl, to standing, then toddle before learning to walk and run.

Life from birth, from the very beginning, is about movement. That movement in itself is an exploration, a discovery. It's not a smooth and linear process, but a series of up and downs, falls and knocks.

'Why do we do anything?' was the question I asked, and then, in the most unexpected way, I found an answer that made sense. We are hardwired to move, to grow, to be inquisitive, and, in an ideal world, through that process follow our interests and passions. Yet not every child is given the opportunity to do so. This insight took me full circle to one of the items in my vision, the 'School of Hope'.

Life is movement, and movement is exploration, and exploration is a service for a greater cause.

I realised, with the help of a practitioner, that in my lack of motion, I could still move, no matter how little that was. With a fuller and deeper breathing pattern, I could lift my rib cage, and in the process bring movements to large parts of my body. I could pull various faces to move my facial muscles. I might not have been able to walk for long periods, but I could circle my feet while sitting down. There were endless motions to carry out. It required patience.

And so it became movement of the mind, which can fuel exploration: to think, to take an idea, to share, to serve a greater cause. When I think of Stephen Hawking, I am always in awe and inspired by what is possible through the human mind, even if movement is restricted.

# EXERCISE: A SIMPLE MOVEMENT EXERCISE THROUGH BREATHING

Disclaimer: Always check with your doctor before taking up any exercise

I want you to either stand or sit facing a mirror. As you look into it, scan your body. What do you notice?

- Now I want you to take a deep breath. What do you notice?

- I want you to carry on with the breathing

- What body parts are moving?

- With each inhalation, do your ribs rise?

- What about your shoulders?

- Whether you are sitting or standing, what's happening to your arms and hands?

Through this small exercise, I want to demonstrate that movement can be achieved through the simple process of breathing. We breathe unconsciously throughout the day, and so we are moving without awareness. By applying attention and intention to the simplest of processes we are able to begin an exploration of movement. I have found this exploration fascinating.

If you want to explore movement further, have a look for Qi Gong or Tai Chi classes. I also participated in gentle yoga classes specifically organised for cancer patients.

In Lesson 2, I shared the story of working with Chris, the movement therapist, after I developed shoulder and knee pain. As I continued to work with Chris, he noticed that I wasn't breathing fully. He encouraged me to breathe all the way to fill my diaphragm. By doing this I began activating and engaging my ribs. When I stood upright, with my arms by my side, the same deep breathing lifted my arms naturally, as well as my upper body and shoulders. More than two years on from my operation, my core abdominal muscles were not being activated, but a simple breathing practice helped engage dormant muscle groups.

# LIFE IS DIFFICULT, IT NEVER GETS EASIER

*'Once we truly know that life is difficult
– once we truly understand and accept it –
then life is no longer difficult. Because once
it is accepted, the fact that life is difficult no
longer matters.'*
**M. Scott Peck**

As I delved into the story of my life as a part of my heal-ing, one thing became clear: there had been many chal-lenges. Each challenge built my character, allowed me to learn certain skills and, in the process, pick up knowledge and make new connections, including long-term friends, teachers and mentors.

When I ran for the students' union elections in 2004 at the age of 21, I barely knew anyone in the union. I was running against the incumbent president and my chanc-es were slim. Yet a voice inside me told me to go for it because I thought I could add value. Speaking to a few trusted friends I decided to go ahead. Doing so meant going into the unknown. I put together a manifesto of what I wanted to do, created posters and leaflets and gave public speeches.

I had to ask people I didn't know to vote for me, which was daunting. When I first spoke into a microphone I almost fainted. I heard one of the students shout 'first aid', as the organiser came with a glass of water. It was a moment when I contemplated quitting, right at the start, but I persevered and got elected.

As the year continued, the challenges intensified. The scrutiny from students was at unexpected levels and once more I thought about walking away. I had written my resignation letter but it was my friend Dave who said: 'Mo, if you run away from this, you'll be running your entire life.' I stayed on and faced a motion on 'no confidence'.

Yet it was these experiences that resulted in my learning more about myself and set me on a trajectory to become more confident and carve out a career path.

Fast forward to the age of 33, and once more I was standing in front of audiences I did not know, speaking through a microphone. This time I wasn't asking for votes, I was asking for money, for prayers and any form of support to help keep me alive. I was talking to politicians, to journalists, I was on TV, on the radio, I attended both small and large events, and I was putting all my previous experiences into this latest chapter of my life.

All the previous layers of challenges had prepared me for this, the biggest challenge. The balance I had to find between new ways of being, compared to my old habits, was tested to the core.

I needed to be real and authentic, as opposed to hiding my inner thoughts. I needed to speak the truth. My previous self would have been conscious about what others thought if I spoke my truth, and would have shied away.

I needed to know what help I required and then be able to ask for that help without being attached to an outcome. I needed to be in a place where hearing a 'no' was an okay response.

If the help was forthcoming, I needed to learn to accept the help. Previously, I would have been reluctant to expose myself to the levels of help I needed and would have feared the rejection.

I needed to let go of perfectionism. I didn't have time to waste getting the video and poster perfect, I just needed to get the message out there. Previously, I would have waited to make sure everything was perfect and acted at the last possible moment, causing unnecessary stress and wasting time. Time was something I didn't have.

I needed to let go of projecting the potential outcomes. I needed to set my intention and act, without being attached to the result. Previously I would have created all sorts of scripts of possible outcomes and played out scenarios which would have been detrimental to my actions.

I also had to act quickly on ideas and 'to do' lists, so there was no time to procrastinate. This was now a case of life and death, any delay could have proved fatal.

To help me with all these new ways of being, I had to remind myself regularly that I was enough, that I was worthy and that I was deserving.

I remembered my vision every day.

I would wake up with a thank you, and go to sleep with a thank you.

I'd have many things to be grateful for during the day.

And when something upset me, I had no time to dwell on it. I would honour the feeling, vent it, process it and then let it go.

There were occasions when I wasn't sure of healthy ways of venting the frustration, but then it became about learning healthy ways of complaining.

## EXERCISE: OVERCOMING CHALLENGES

- What are some of the biggest challenges you have faced?

- Are there similarities between them?

- Are there patterns?

- What did you learn?

- Who did you meet as a result?

- What new skills, behaviours and habits did you develop that have improved your life?

- Did life take a new trajectory as a result of the challenges?

- What positives/benefits did you experience?

Use all these learnings and integrate them for your next challenge.

I feel extremely lucky that I have had so much support from my family, friends, mentors, the community and from complete strangers, many of whom are close friends now. Yet with that luck I realise I've had to take important lessons from previous experiences and build on those to put myself out there.

I was ready to be seen, to be heard, to be vulnerable and to share my story, and I was prepared to be rejected again. The NHS said no, the drug companies said no, the Department for Health said no. But I said yes, and so did Team Mo, to whom I am indebted.

If my premise is that the challenges will continue, then I can expect more opportunities to venture out of my comfort zone. Instead of fearing the challenges, I will embrace them knowing that previous layers have held me in good stead. The cycle will no doubt continue.

As I write this book, I am asking myself psychological and emotional questions. Is what I'm writing relevant? Will anyone want to read it? Am I sharing too much information?

All I know is that I am sharing my life publicly once more, more intimately, to an audience over whom I have no control. I am pouring out my heart and soul with a deep yearning to add value to your life.

# LIFE IS A MASTERPIECE – CONNECT THE DOTS

*'You can't connect the dots looking forward; you can only connect them looking backward. So you have to trust that the dots will somehow connect in your future. You have to trust in something – your gut, destiny, life, karma, whatever.'*
**Steve Jobs**

I truly believe our lives are masterpieces. I believe life is fascinating. When I take myself out of my life and look back, I am in awe.

One Saturday morning in 1998, when I was fifteen, I walked into my newsagent to buy a newspaper in the hope that there was cash inside a moneybag promotion. Instead of winning the cash, I was offered a job. I started work the following week. Not only was I earning money and experiencing a commercial environment, which would help me later in my career, I was getting first-hand life experience. I was meeting people from various backgrounds and ages, with different levels of wealth and experiences, and through that I was gaining invaluable knowledge. I was also getting the chance to be independent. I was earning, saving and buying my own things, as well as presents for others.

While working in the shop, I met David, a regular customer, with whom I am still in regular contact. David is one of my trusted mentors and guides my breathwork sessions, which are part of my self-care practice. He has also, throughout the last 20 years helped me explore various themes and patterns in my life, facilitating awareness and healthier behaviours.

I look back and see how not getting the grades to go to my first choice university led me to go to Middlesex University, which then resulted in my finding an unusual career path. It was through this Middlesex connection that I met Leonard, who has become a long-term friend, mentor and another wise person. The challenges in the students' union resulted in my discovering personal development, which then became a huge resource for me when cancer became my reality.

It was during my life examination that I went through old journals and notepads and remembered an encounter I had with a shaman who was over from Zimbabwe. I was twenty five at the time and was introduced to Colin by another one of my mentors. The shaman had a bag of stones and bones and threw them onto a mat in front of me. He said that I would go through a huge challenge during the ages of twenty nine and thirty three and that at the ages of thirty four and thirty five I would develop a deep spiritual base. After that I would take all my learning and experiences and go on and be of service to the world. I had completely forgotten that encounter until I began searching for my life's meaning. Seeing the notes from that session was overwhelming. I was diagnosed at thirty-one, told the cancer was terminal at thirty-two, and then I began fundraising at thirty-three for a potentially life-saving drug. I was thirty-four when I began to document my experiences and learnings for this book. I am thirty-five as I come to the end of writing this book. I remain detached about how things will unfold, but looking back over the story is fascinating.

I've written about my dad dying, 'the curse' story that has passed down my family for generations, my fears of losing my mum and my desire to work with orphans and street kids from a very young age. The personal development books that led me to several teachers and mentors, as well as all the students who have come my way, many of whom are close friends – everything is connected.

It was Steve Jobs in his Stanford commencement address who said: 'You can only connect the dots looking backward.'

I don't know how the future will pan out, but I do know the dots are being created in the moment. Every day there are choices, choices to make such as: to be still, to move, to be quiet, to listen, to act, to speak, to follow our intuition, to either stay in a comfort zone or take a step into the unknown, to acknowledge fear and to trust, to be real, to be ready to be wrong, to be ready to say yes. Every day, there are new dots being plotted, and at some point in the future we can look back and see the masterpiece that our lives really are.

## EXERCISE: CONNECTING YOUR DOTS

I invite you to look back at your dots, to go on an exploration to find those dots, to plot them, to connect them and to create new dots. As Jobs says: 'to trust that the dots will connect.'

The process is rewarding and liberating.

I would then encourage you to be conscious of each new day you have.

- What new dots can you start plotting now?

- What ideas do you have?

- Who have you stalled in connecting with?

Are you waiting for a perfect moment? Are you waiting for the right way? Perhaps you are waiting for permission from an authority figure?

'It's never the right time, and there's never a right way,' are words a mentor once said.

'So you might as well just get on with it with the best way you know.'

Procrastination won't plot those new dots. No doubt that by getting on with it, you will get feedback and learn better ways.

Remember this is your life, and you have so much value within. My wish and hope is for you to see that value if you don't already and live the rest of your life with the feeling of liberation.

In 2012, when I went to see Gabby B live in London, I would never have known that 'choosing to stay' would be three important words for me, let alone the title of this book. It was a random question from the audience that I remember from that talk. Looking back, I remember having a number of reasons not to go to the event but after listening to that inner voice I decided to turn up.

Cancer has given me a new set of principles to live my life by, which I've laid out in this book. It breaks my heart when someone tells me they are about to start chemotherapy.

I hope there comes a day when nobody has to go through the devastating effects of cancer.

The reality, when we look at the trends and the data, is that many more people will get the disease unfortunately.

There are people working to eradicate all diseases, but the time scale for this is one hundred years. What do we do now? I would love there to be a time when a doctor says, 'It's cancer,' and the patient responds, without any fear: 'Okay, what options do we have?' A time when cancer is nothing serious and can just be seen and treated in the same way as a common cold.

# A BRAVE NEW LIFE

It is difficult to remember the specifics of what life was like before cancer entered my consciousness. When someone asks me about my pre-cancer world, I struggle. I do not know if there will be a post-cancer world, but in the realm of possibility that could be a reality. At the moment the tumours are stable and I nervously go from scan to scan. There are niggles, there are scares, and then there are always the little things to remind me how amazing life is.

If there's one message I want you to take from this book it's that life is sacred.

None of us can escape death, the cycle that completes birth, but life is a thread that is part of a continuum, even in a serious diagnosis such as terminal cancer

Cancer has changed me, and it has given me a totally new outlook on life.

Life is fleeting and, as The Beatles say in one of their songs: 'Life is very short and there's no time for fussing and fighting, my friend.'

I appreciate those words more than I ever would have done prior to my diagnosis.

Before cancer, I was sabotaged with the evil 'P's: perfectionism, projection, procrastination and people-pleasing. Now, I live each day true to my values and vision, and appreciate and honour myself before anyone else. That's why I say 'cancer gave me my life back'. And it is in this vein that I hope to go on and be of service to humanity, however that manifests itself.

I am humbled, grateful and genuinely lucky to be writing these words. I am thankful to everyone who has played a part in #TeamMo. I love you all.

There is not a day that goes by when I do not think about death. Sometimes it's when I go to bed, sometimes it's when I wake up, and sometimes it's during my waking hours. I've even had times when I've dreamed about dying and being prepared for my funeral.

I've accepted that I will die, one day. The appreciation that death is the opposite of birth, and life is what cuts through, gives me comfort. I often remember those who have left us here on the physical plane and the words of Persian poet and Sufi master Rumi are always comforting: 'When I die to the body I shall soar with the angels, when I die to the angels what I shall become, you cannot imagine.'

I pray for life every day. I pray for more time, time to create more moments, to appreciate the little things and to work on 'my picture'.

Healing is my life full time now; I am always looking for ways to helps others. I've been honoured to speak on different stages and have been featured on various media platforms. I am working with different charities to raise awareness about cancer, to campaign for access and to do preventative work.

I've come to the end of this book, and dare I say a theme for a second book has emerged.

For anyone who wants to know more about the specifics of my fundraising, I have put together a guide, The Price On Life, which can be downloaded from www.mohaque.com.

Wherever you are in life, I hope that through reading my story you will be able to get closer to making the choices that feel right for you. I thank you for giving me your time and energy, and it is my deep wish to have been of value in some small way.

All my love,

Mo

# ACKNOWLEDGEMENTS

Dr Kim Jobst, your words still resonate with me: 'Mo, you are more powerful than the words of any doctor.' You have walked with me every step of the way since. Meanings definitely matter.

Dr Pelz, Jacquie Peck, Mr McCullough, Professor Bridgewater, Dr Tobias Arkenau, Sam Hughes: there have been bad days, and then the unimaginably dark ones. Your support, expertise and dedication in what you do have helped me through many tough times – you are truly world class.

David Parker: I didn't know at the age of 15 in 1998 that you would become my friend and mentor for the next 20 years, and I hope for many more. You inspire me, and always remind me to take one breath at a time.

Leonard Daniels: your friendship, wisdom and ear for the psychosomatic make all the difference.

Jack Turner: you've been a neighbour all my life, but through cancer you've become a true friend. I am blessed to know you.

Jean-Pierre De Villiers: you believed in me from our first phone call and gave me my first speaking opportunity. Two years on, and my first book is here!

Chopper: you've been fixing my hair since I was a kid, but you've also been listening to all my troubles (and those of Spurs!) for over 25 years. We somehow still have hair, even after the chemo.

Daljeet Singh, Chris Sritharan and Anastasia Hatzivasilou: you all helped me explore my mind, body and soul to deeper levels.

Maha Khan: wherever in the world you happen to be I know you're just a message away, whether that's to proof something, give me a second medical opinion, or to hear me ramble on about something pointless. You have kept me sane through some crazy times.

Roberta Ramos and David Medawar: we have come a long way from our student union officer days to now. What do you say?

Joy Zarine: the words in this book would not have been written if it hadn't been for your encouragement and brutal honesty. You once said, 'the world can't wait for you to be ready.' I'm still not ready, but here goes anyway.

Lucy McCarraher, Joe Gregory and the Rethink Press team: your kindness, patience and support to publish this book have overwhelmed me. Outside my fundraising, this has been the most daunting thing I have attempted. You have taken away all the hassle.

Marc Garcia: I was nervous about the thought of a cover shoot. You put me at ease and captured the perfect photos.

Daniel Priestley: you have brought together some of the world's finest thought leaders and key people of influence through your team at Dent, so many of whom are part of my healing. I aspire to be one of those influencers.

Saiful Abdin and Ruhel Mohammed: outside of my family you boys have known me longer than anyone. When you heard of my cancer you became family.

Kayes Ahmed and the team at Up My Street: you guys provide me with an office, distract me from my cancer story, give me a break from the hospital, all the while entertaining me with your hospitality.

Aadam Ali – dude! You began as my protégé but very soon became my best friend.

Dasha Saini: I continue to test your patience. Keep smiling.

Charlie Hudson: you continue to be there, your Kingston students continue to be there.

Rui Daniel Jaime: you keep me believing anything is possible.

Nicola Skevington: you saw me in pain day after day before my diagnosis, and when I could no longer go into work, you always stayed in touch.

Alex and Stephanie: your 50-day bike trek across New Zealand scared me, but wow – you did it!

Keir Starmer MP: not only did you represent me but you looked for ways to spread the message. I will never ever forget the reception you hosted for me in Parliament.

I am also forever indebted to:

- Sheikh Madani for instilling my duty to seek treatment

- my local community in Camden, who rallied

- all the mosques that ran collections

Sincere thanks to:

- Rizwan Hussain and TV One

- Abu Taher and Bangla TV

- Farhan Khan, Tauhidul Mujahid and Channel S

- Shab Uddin, Forhad Tipu and The Beani Bazar Cancer & General Hospital

You all gave me a platform on live television and campaigned vigorously for me. I have no words.

To #TeamMo: It's impossible to include every name as there are thousands of people who have contributed and continue to be with me. You all prove that humanity is still alive. I wouldn't still be here if it wasn't for you, I love you all.

A huge thank you to the various media outlets for covering my campaign: ITV London News, the Evening Standard, the Ham & High, the Camden New Journal, The Independent, talkRADIO, and the Eastern Eye.

My family: cousins, sister and brother in laws, uncles and aunts, all extending throughout the world, thank you.

Uncle Zuel: I remember reading the news to you as a child, and then all these years later we find ourselves making the news in between hospital visits and the fundraising.

My sister Shereen, and brother Nazmul: you put up with me as the baby of the family, and three decades later I'm still making you both look out for me.

Lastly Amma (Mum): you've always been there unconditionally for me, whatever the time, whatever the situation, whatever the challenge, and you've been right about most things. You've taught me always to find a way.

… and Dad: I finally got to know you.

# THE AUTHOR

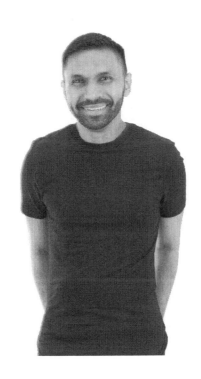

Mo Haque unexpectedly became a cancer patient in 2014. Having spent over ten years in personal and student development, Mo approached his diagnosis with vulnerability, authenticity and a search for meaning.

He raised £190,000 for a new experimental drug after the health system could no longer provide him with any treatment, and, as a result, has seen his cancer reduce and stabilise.

Mo now provides guidance to other patients who are embarking on similar crowdfunding journeys for treatment. He is a patient advocate, features in publications and in the media, and also shares his insights at industry conferences and events.

Mo has a passion for people empowerment, and is applying his previous professional experience to the cancer space, to help patients find their voice in what can be a daunting process. His mission is to empower patients to liberate their lives.

Mo believes the cancer landscape is changing rapidly with new advancements in science, but access to drugs can be a huge barrier. He wants his story to help pave the way for others to get access to life-saving treatment.

www.mohaque.com
Twitter: @momenulhaque

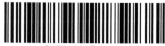
31771807R00103

Printed in Great Britain
by Amazon